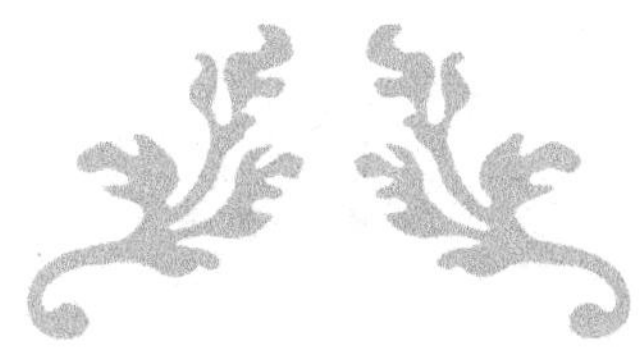

PULSE OF LIFE: THE ART AND SCIENCE OF NADI PARIKSHAN

Decoding Ancient Rhythms for Today's Wellness Revolution

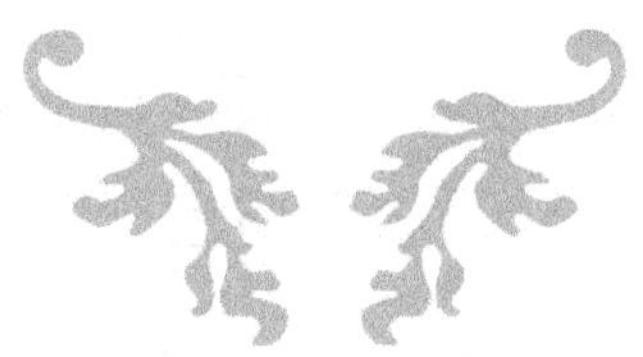

DR VIVEK SINGH
BAMS, MD(AYU), PGDCRPV, PHD (SCH)
ASSISTANT PROFESSOR AND AYURVEDA
PRACTITIONER

Index

<u>Preface</u>

The journey of understanding and perfecting the art of Nadi Parikshan has been nothing short of extraordinary. As both an ancient healing practice and a profound diagnostic tool, pulse examination offers a gateway into the rich tapestry of Ayurveda—a holistic system of medicine that has guided the well-being of countless generations. Writing Pulse of Life: The Art and Science of Nadi Parikshan has been a deeply personal endeavour, inspired by years of study, practice, and an unwavering belief in the constructive collaboration between ancient wisdom and modern medical insights.

The decision to draft this book stemmed from a growing realization: the timeless principles of Ayurveda possess an unmatched potential to enrich contemporary healthcare practices. Nadi Parikshan is a testament to the depth and intricacy of Ayurvedic diagnostics, offering insights into the balance and imbalance of the tridoshas—Vata, Pitta, and Kapha—which govern our physiological and psychological states.

Throughout my career, I have witnessed the transformative power of pulse diagnosis. From uncovering subtle imbalances to providing a roadmap for personalized treatment, Nadi

Parikshan has proven to be an invaluable guide for practitioners and patients alike. This book is a compilation of those experiences, intertwined with an earnest attempt to present both the traditional aspects and the latest research in pulse study.

In this era of unprecedented advancements in medical science, it is crucial to encourage a dialogue between ancient practices and modern technologies. Through this book, I hope to demonstrate how Nadi Parikshan can seamlessly integrate with contemporary diagnostic methods, creating a more comprehensive and patient-cantered approach to health and wellness.

The chapters that follow will take you on a journey through the foundational principles of Ayurveda, the intricate science of pulse examination, and the exciting possibilities of integrating these with current medical practices. You will find discussions enriched with case studies, practical applications, and future directions that aim to inspire practitioners and lay readers alike.

As I present Pulse of Life: The Art and Science of Nadi Parikshan to you, my hope is that it ignites a curiosity to explore the harmonious blend of ancient and modern healing, fostering a new paradigm of wellness that honours our past and embraces our future.

In gratitude,
Dr Vivek B Singh
BAMS, MD(Ayu), PGDCRPV, PhD (Sch)

Foreword

It is with immense pleasure and reverence that I introduce Pulse of Life: The Art and Science of Nadi Parikshan, a remarkable work authored by Dr Vivek Singh, a distinguished practitioner and scholar in the field of Ayurveda. This book is a profound contribution to the understanding and practice of Nadi Parikshan, an art that has fascinated healers for centuries and continues to offer invaluable insights into human health and wellness.

My acquaintance with Dr Vivek began many years ago, when we first shared conversations about the intricate balances and rhythms that define life itself. Over time, I have had the privilege of witnessing their relentless dedication to mastering this ancient practice. It is a rare individual who successfully bridges the gap between ancient wisdom and the demands of modern healthcare. Dr Vivek is one such individual, passionately committed to enhancing the discourse between these disparate worlds.

In the pages of this book, you will discover the profound depths of Ayurvedic knowledge, meticulously woven into practical applications that are relevant to today's practitioners. Dr Vivek has deftly navigated the historical context and foundational theories of Nadi Parikshan while elegantly introducing modern scientific perspectives that can complement this ancient practice. This fusion opens new pathways for understanding the human body and mind, offering a comprehensive approach to diagnosis and wellness.

One of the most commendable aspects of this work is its accessible style, ensuring that the knowledge contained within is not only reserved for seasoned practitioners but is also available to anyone with a genuine interest in holistic health. Whether you are a curious reader, an aspiring Ayurvedic practitioner, or an established healthcare professional, there is much to gain from the insights shared in this book.

It is my sincere belief that Pulse of Life: The Art and Science of Nadi Parikshan will serve as an invaluable resource and inspiration to all who are in pursuit of integrating traditional wisdom with modern science. Dr Vivek has gifted us with a profound reminder of the interconnectedness of all life, a reminder that is needed now more than ever.

I invite you to embark on this journey with an open heart and mind, and I am confident that you will emerge with a deeper appreciation for the pulse that unites us all.

With warm regards,
Dr Abhijit Patil
BAMS, MD
Professor and HOD, Sharir Rachna Dept,
RKCAMS, Bhopal.

Introduction to Ayurveda

Ayurveda, often referred to as the "science of life," is one of the world's oldest holistic healing systems, originating in India over 5,000 years ago. It is a comprehensive approach to health and well-being that goes beyond merely treating symptoms to address the root causes of imbalance or disease.

At its core, Ayurveda teaches that health is not just the absence of illness but a balance of the body, mind, and spirit with nature and the cosmos. The word "Ayurveda" itself is derived from the Sanskrit words "ayur" meaning life and "veda" meaning knowledge or science. This ancient science provides a roadmap to living life in harmony with the laws of nature, emphasizing the preventive and curative aspects of health.

The Foundational Concepts

Ayurveda is built upon several foundational concepts, with the central tenet being the Tridosha theory—Vata, Pitta, and Kapha. These are the three biological energies or doshas that govern all physical and mental processes. Everyone has a unique constitution, or Prakriti, determined by the dominance of these doshas, which affects everything from physical characteristics to personality traits and predisposition to diseases.

1. Vata: This dosha is associated with the elements of air and space. It governs movement, communication, and flexibility within the body and mind. Vata is considered the force behind all biological activity, influencing everything from circulation to breathing.

2. Pitta: Linked to fire and water elements, Pitta is responsible for transformation processes, including digestion, metabolism, and energy production. It is also associated with mental functions like intelligence and comprehension.

3. Kapha: Comprised of earth and water elements, Kapha provides structure, stability, and lubrication. It governs growth, tissue formation, and the retention of energy.

The Role of Prakriti and Vikriti

Understanding an individual's Prakriti helps tailor lifestyle and treatment plans to maintain balance, as deviations from the Prakriti result in Vikriti, or imbalances, often leading to disease. Ayurvedic practices are thus highly personalized, recognizing the uniqueness of everyone.

The Importance of Agni and Ojas

Ayurveda also emphasizes the significance of Agni, the digestive fire, crucial for proper digestion, absorption, and assimilation of nutrients. Balanced Agni is essential for health, while impaired Agni is a root cause of disease. Ojas, the essence of immunity and vitality, is another critical component in maintaining health, providing the body with strength and resilience against illnesses.

Holistic and Integrative Approaches

The holistic nature of Ayurveda encompasses not only physical aspects but also mental and spiritual dimensions. Practices such as yoga, meditation, and pranayama (breathing exercises) are integral to promoting mental clarity and spiritual growth. Additionally, Ayurveda encourages the use of natural remedies, diet, seasonal routines, detoxification practices, and ethical living principles to sustain balance and health.

In recent years, Ayurveda has gained global recognition for its integrative and preventive approach to health. It offers valuable insights and practices that complement modern medical advancements, thereby enriching the global healthcare system.

As you delve into the profound world of Ayurveda, you are invited to explore the interconnectedness of life and the wisdom that has endured through millennia, promising a harmonious way to health and well-being.

The Significance of Nadi Parikshan in Ayurveda

Nadi Parikshan, or pulse examination, is a cornerstone of diagnostic techniques in Ayurveda, embodying the profound depth and precision of this ancient system of medicine. The significance of Nadi Parikshan lies in its ability to offer a comprehensive understanding of an individual's health, transcending mere symptoms to reveal subtle physiological and psychological imbalances.

The Heartbeat of Diagnosis

In Ayurveda, the pulse is regarded as a mirror of the body's internal state, reflecting the dynamic balance of the tridoshas—Vata, Pitta, and Kapha. By examining the pulse, a skilled practitioner can infer the constitution (Prakriti) of an individual, and more importantly, discern imbalances (Vikriti) that may predispose to or indicate existing ailments. This diagnostic method empowers practitioners to create personalized treatment plans that restore balance and promote holistic health.

A Subtle Art

Nadi Parikshan is often considered an art form, requiring years of study, practice, and intuition. Practitioners develop sensitivity to the distinct qualities associated with each dosha, such as the quick and irregular pulse of Vata, the strong and bounding pulse of Pitta, and the slow and steady pulse of Kapha. Additionally, they learn to identify the subtle variations and combinations that indicate complex health issues or the involvement of specific organs and tissues.

Comprehensive Health Insight

The reach of Nadi Parikshan extends far beyond determining dosha imbalances. It can provide insights into the health and functioning of the seven bodily tissues (dhatus), the presence of toxins (ama), and the efficiency of the digestive fire (Agni). Moreover, it reflects the state of one's mental and emotional health, offering clues to conditions that might not have yet manifested physically.

Preventive and Curative Power

One of the most remarkable aspects of Nadi Parikshan is its preventive potential. By identifying imbalances before they manifest as disease, practitioners can recommend lifestyle and dietary modifications, herbal remedies, or detoxification procedures like Panchakarma. This preemptive approach aligns perfectly with Ayurveda's emphasis on prevention and individualized care.

Bridging Ancient and Modern

In today's world, the wisdom of Nadi Parikshan is finding new resonance as it begins to align with and influence modern diagnostic methodologies. By incorporating insights from modern pulse analysis techniques, Ayurveda can broaden its applications and interface with contemporary healthcare paradigms.

The Path to Mastery

While the practice of Nadi Parikshan demands diligence and expertise, it is also a rewarding pursuit that enhances the practitioner's ability to provide deeply personalized care. Training involves developing an acute sensitivity to the nuances of the pulse and an understanding of the broader context of Ayurvedic physiology and pathology.

Nadi Parikshan stands as a testament to the intricacy and insight of Ayurvedic diagnostics. Its ability to integrate physiological, psychological, and spiritual dimensions of health makes it an invaluable tool for practitioners and patients seeking comprehensive health solutions. By acknowledging the significance of Nadi Parikshan, we embrace a deeper understanding of the human experience and the holistic vision of Ayurveda.

Objectives of the Book

Pulse of Life: The Art and Science of Nadi Parikshan aims to serve as a comprehensive guide and resource for both practitioners and enthusiasts of Ayurveda. The objectives of this book are multi-faceted, seeking to deepen the understanding of Nadi Parikshan while exploring its integration with modern medical practices. Here is what this book intends to achieve:

1. Illuminate the Foundations of Nadi Parikshan:
   - To provide a thorough exploration of the historical and theoretical underpinnings of pulse examination in Ayurveda, highlighting its role and evolution over centuries.

2. Enhance Diagnostic Proficiency:
   - To equip readers with the knowledge and skills necessary to accurately assess the pulse, recognizing the unique signatures of Vata, Pitta, and Kapha doshas, as well as their combinations and imbalances.

3. Bridge Ancient and Modern Practices:

- To explore the intersection of ancient Ayurvedic methods and contemporary medical science, demonstrating how Nadi Parikshan can be complemented by modern diagnostic tools for a more holistic approach to health.

4. Promote Holistic Health and Personalized Care:

 - To underscore the importance of personalized treatment plans based on pulse diagnosis, emphasizing Ayurveda's preventive and curative strategies for maintaining optimal health.

5. Share Practical Applications and Case Studies:

 - To present a variety of real-world case studies and practical applications, showcasing the versatility and efficacy of Nadi Parikshan in diagnosing and treating various health conditions.

6. Encourage the Integration of Ayurveda in Modern Healthcare:

 - To advocate for the inclusion of Ayurvedic practices, particularly Nadi Parikshan, in mainstream healthcare settings by providing evidence and insights into its effectiveness.

7. Facilitate Skill Development:

 - To guide aspiring practitioners on the path to mastering pulse diagnosis, offering resources for further study, training pathways, and ethical considerations in practice.

8. Inspire Research and Innovation:

 - To stimulate interest in further research and innovation within the field of Nadi Parikshan, inviting collaboration between Ayurvedic practitioners and scientific researchers to expand its scope and potential.

By achieving these objectives, this book seeks to be a definitive resource for those committed to understanding and applying Nadi Parikshan as part of a holistic approach to health and healing. It invites readers to embrace the rich traditions of Ayurveda while engaging with the possibilities offered by modern advancements, crafting a future of integrative wellness.

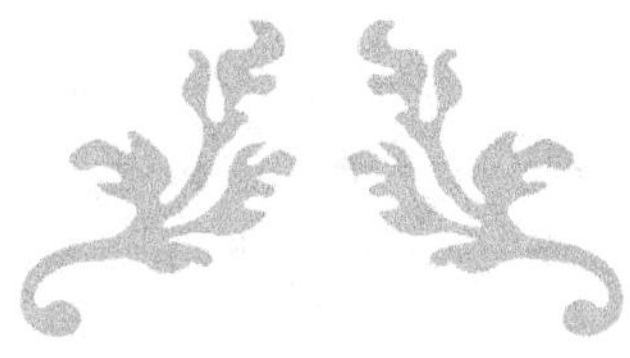

CHAPTER 1 – FUNDAMENTALS OF AYURVEDA

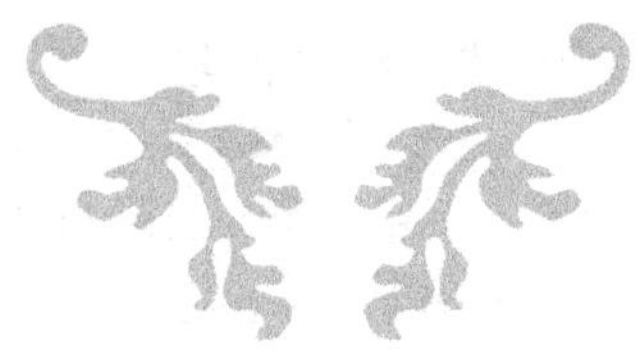

1.1 The Principles of Ayurveda

Ayurveda, often described as the "science of life," encompasses a vast body of knowledge designed to guide individuals toward optimal health and well-being. Rooted in the belief that health results from the harmonious balance of mind, body, and spirit, Ayurveda provides a comprehensive framework for understanding and achieving this balance. Here are the foundational principles that underpin this ancient system of medicine:

Holistic Health Approach

Ayurveda views health as a dynamic and holistic state of balance across the physical, mental, emotional, and spiritual dimensions of life. Rather than focusing solely on treating symptoms, it aims to address the root causes of imbalance, promoting lasting wellness through a personalized and integrative approach.

The Tridosha Theory

At the heart of Ayurvedic philosophy is the concept of the three doshas: Vata, Pitta, and Kapha. These are the fundamental energies or bio-energetic forces that govern all physiological and psychological processes within the body:

- **Vata:** Comprised of the elements of air and space (ether), Vata governs movement, communication, and the nervous system. It influences activities like breathing, circulation, and elimination.

- **Pitta:** Made up of the elements of fire and water, Pitta is responsible for metabolic processes, including digestion, absorption, and temperature regulation. It also encompasses qualities like intelligence and courage.

- **Kapha:** Formed from earth and water elements, Kapha provides structure, stability, and lubrication to the body and mind. It influences growth, tissue integrity, and emotional calmness.

Each individual has a unique constitution or Prakriti, determined by the balance of these doshas at the time of conception. Understanding one's Prakriti is crucial for maintaining health and designing personalized lifestyle and treatment plans.

The Concept of Prakriti and Vikriti

Prakriti, the natural constitution of an individual, remains constant throughout life, while Vikriti represents the current state of dosha imbalance. Ayurveda focuses on restoring balance by addressing Vikriti, tailoring interventions to the individual's unique constitution and current condition.

The Role of Agni

Agni, the digestive fire, is crucial for the transformation and assimilation of food and experiences. Balanced Agni supports proper digestion, absorption, and elimination, playing a key role in health. When Agni is impaired, it leads to the accumulation of toxins (ama) and disease.

The Importance of the Dhatus and Malas

Ayurveda recognizes the seven dhatus, or bodily tissues, and their roles in maintaining structure and function. These include the physical tissues (Rasa, Rakta, Mamsa, Meda, Asthi, Majja, and Shukra) and the Malas (waste products), which need to be balanced for optimal health.

Focus on Prevention and Longevity

Prevention is a cornerstone of Ayurvedic philosophy, emphasizing lifestyle and dietary practices that align with one's Prakriti, seasonal changes, and environmental factors. By fostering balance and preventing disease, Ayurveda aims for a long, healthy life characterized by vitality and well-being.

Integration with the Cosmos

Ayurveda teaches that individuals are an integral part of the universe, and the same elements and principles that govern nature also affect human health. Understanding this interconnectedness is key to living in harmony with nature and achieving a balanced, healthy life.

Through these guiding principles, Ayurveda offers a timeless and profound path to health and wellness, encouraging individuals to take an active role in their healing journeys by aligning themselves with the inherent rhythms and laws of nature.

1.2 The Tridosha Theory: Vata, Pitta, and Kapha

The Tridosha Theory is a fundamental concept in Ayurveda, explaining how three primary energies—Vata, Pitta, and Kapha— govern all biological, psychological, and physio pathological functions of the body, mind, and consciousness. These doshas are the forces behind individual constitution and the core pillars of health and disease processes in Ayurveda.

Vata Dosha

- Composed of: Air and Space (Ether) elements.
- Qualities: Dry, light, cold, rough, subtle, mobile, and clear.

Functions:

Vata is the dynamic force that governs movement and communication within the body. It is responsible for all muscular and tissue activity, nerve conduction, breathing, circulation, elimination, and even the movement of thoughts and emotions.

Imbalance Symptoms:
When Vata is balanced, creativity and flexibility flourish; when unbalanced, it can lead to fear, anxiety, and physical symptoms like dry skin, irregular digestion, insomnia, and joint pain.

Pitta Dosha
- Composed of: Fire and Water elements.
- Qualities: Hot, sharp, light, oily, liquid, and sour.

Functions:
Pitta governs transformation and metabolism in the body. It influences digestion, absorption, assimilation, nutrition, metabolism, and temperature regulation. Pitta also plays a critical role in mental functions, contributing to intelligence, courage, and determination.

Imbalance Symptoms:
A balanced Pitta results in contentment and intellect, but when imbalanced, it can lead to anger, irritation, inflammation, and disorders such as heartburn, skin rashes, and ulcers.

Kapha Dosha
- Composed of: Earth and Water elements.
- Qualities: Heavy, slow, steady, solid, cold, soft, and oily.

Functions:

Kapha is the energy of growth and maintenance, providing structure, strength, and lubrication to the body and mind. It governs the formation of tissues and bones and provides emotional support through stability and calm.

Imbalance Symptoms:
Balance in Kapha leads to love, patience, and forgiveness; imbalance can cause lethargy, weight gain, congestion, and conditions like diabetes, depression, and allergies.

Balancing the Doshas
Each person has a unique combination of these three doshas, which defines their constitution, or Prakriti. The dynamic balance among the doshas both within oneself and between oneself and the environment determines health and wellness. Disruptions to this balance, or Vikriti, can result from factors like stress, unhealthy diet, seasonal changes, and other lifestyle mismatches, leading to various health issues.

Using the Tridosha Theory in Practice
Understanding the Tridosha Theory allows Ayurvedic practitioners to tailor health interventions precisely. These may include specific dietary recommendations, herbal remedies, therapies like Panchakarma, and lifestyle adjustments designed to restore balance. For instance:

- To pacify Vata, one might focus on stability with warm, moist foods, calming routines, and grounding practices.
- To balance Pitta, cooling foods, stress reduction, and soothing activities are emphasized.
- To alleviate Kapha imbalances, invigorating diets and exercises along with cleansing treatments are recommended.

By respecting and harmonizing the distinctive energies of Vata, Pitta, and Kapha, Ayurveda provides a personalized road map to health, underscoring its philosophy that prevention comes from understanding and maintaining balance within the life forces.

1.3 The Concept of Prakriti (Constitution)

Prakriti, which translates to "nature" or "constitution" in Sanskrit, is a core concept in Ayurveda that reflects an individual's unique physical, mental, and emotional characteristics. It is the inherent balance of the tridoshas—Vata, Pitta, and Kapha—established at the time of conception and remains unchanged throughout one's life.

Understanding Prakriti

Prakriti can be thought of as a person's natural state of equilibrium and is determined by numerous factors, including genetics, the diet and lifestyle of the parents, environmental conditions, and even the time and place of conception. While every person possesses all three doshas, they exist in unique proportions that define their Prakriti. This biological blueprint influences a range of characteristics, from body shape and personality traits to metabolic tendencies and health predispositions.

The Role of Prakriti in Health

Prakriti plays a vital role in determining how an individual responds to various internal and external stimuli, and it guides Ayurvedic practitioners in crafting personalized wellness routines. By understanding one's Prakriti, individuals can make informed choices about diet, exercise, work, and relationships, ultimately fostering balance and preventing disease.

Categories of Prakriti

Prakriti is generally categorized into three main types, though mixed types are prevalent:

1. Vata Prakriti:
  - Individuals often exhibit thin builds, dry skin, and high energy levels.
  - They are creative, enthusiastic, and quick to grasp new information but may struggle with anxiety and overexertion.
  - They thrive in warm and stable environments, and benefit from grounding routines and nourishing diets.

2. Pitta Prakriti:
  - These individuals usually have a medium build, fair or reddish skin, and a strong digestion.
  - They are intelligent, ambitious, and passionate but can be prone to anger and impatience.
  - To maintain balance, they should seek cooling foods and environments, and practice stress-relieving activities.

3. Kapha Prakriti:
  - Characterized by a sturdy build, oily skin, and a calm demeanor.
  - They possess great endurance, loyalty, and compassion, but may face issues with weight gain and lethargy.
  - Stimulation through vigorous exercise and lighter meals help maintain their equilibrium.

Prakriti in Disease Prevention and Treatment

Ayurveda emphasizes that maintaining one's Prakriti is key to preventing Vikriti, or imbalance, which can lead to disease. Recognizing one's constitution allows for personalized approaches in both lifestyle and therapeutic interventions. For instance, understanding the imbalances that Pitta individuals are prone to, like inflammatory conditions, they can implement cooling strategies proactively.

The Dynamic Interplay with Vikriti

While Prakriti does not change, Vikriti—the current state of dosha balance—can fluctuate based on lifestyle, diet, stress levels, environment, and other factors. Ayurvedic diagnosis and treatment focus on aligning Vikriti back to one's natural Prakriti, which is considered the state of optimal health.

Practical Insights

Understanding your Prakriti is a step toward self-awareness and empowerment. It encourages mindful living in accordance with one's natural tendencies and environmental context. Ayurvedic practitioners use Prakriti as a diagnostic tool to tailor preventive measures and healing practices that support an individual's unique blueprint for health and vitality.

1.4 The Role of Agni (Digestive Fire)

In Ayurveda, Agni, the Sanskrit word for "fire," is a vital force responsible for all metabolic and transformative processes in the body. It is considered the source of life, health, and vitality, and thus, plays a central role in maintaining and restoring balance. Agni governs digestion, absorption, assimilation, and transformation of food and sensations into energy, shaping both physical health and mental clarity.

The Functions of Agni

- Digestion and Metabolism: Agni facilitates the breakdown of food into nutrients, ensuring proper digestion and nutrient absorption. It converts these nutrients into the essential components needed for maintaining bodily tissues, energy, and vitality.

- Tissue Metabolism: Agni regulates the metabolism of the seven dhatus (bodily tissues), ensuring they receive the nourishment they need to function optimally.

- Mental Clarity and Perception: Beyond physical digestion, Agni is responsible for processing sensory impressions, emotions, and thoughts. A balanced Agni promotes mental acuity, decision-making, and emotional stability.

- Immune Function: Healthy Agni contributes to a robust immune system, forming a potent defence against pathogens and diseases. It supports the production of Ojas, the essence of vitality and immunity.

Types of Agni

Ayurveda describes various types of Agni based on their roles within the body:

1. **Jatharagni**: The central digestive fire located in the stomach and duodenum, responsible for digesting gross food substances.

2. **Bhootagni**: These are five elemental fires that convert the elemental components of digested food into substances that can nourish the tissues.

3. **Dhatwagni**: The seven tissue fires responsible for transforming digested nutrients into bodily tissues (dhatus), such as blood, muscle, and fat.

States of Agni

Maintaining the right state of Agni is crucial for health:

- **Sama Agni (Balanced Digestive Fire)**: Reflects optimal function, promoting efficient digestion, assimilation, and elimination. It indicates strong immunity and vibrant health.

- **Vishama Agni (Irregular Digestive Fire)**: Often associated with Vata imbalance, leading to variable appetite, bloating, gas, and irregular digestion patterns.

- **Tikshna Agni (Intense Digestive Fire)**: Common in Pitta individuals, characterized by strong but excessive appetite and symptoms of acidity, inflammation, and hyper-metabolism.

- **Manda Agni (Dull Digestive Fire)**: Related to Kapha imbalance, resulting in sluggish digestion, loss of appetite, weight gain, and lethargy.

The Importance of Balancing Agni

Balanced Agni is fundamental to preventing and managing disease. An impaired Agni can lead to the accumulation of toxins (Ama), which are considered the root cause of most health issues. Ayurveda provides various strategies to balance Agni and support digestive health:

- Diet and Nutrition: Consuming warm, fresh, and cooked foods suitable for one's dosha type can help maintain Agni.

- Lifestyle Practices: Regular routines, mindfulness in eating, and stress management techniques like meditation and yoga can support Agni.

- Herbal Supplements and Spices: Incorporating certain herbs and spices like ginger, cumin, and turmeric can enhance digestive function.

Agni is a cornerstone of Ayurvedic health, representing the transformative processes essential for maintaining life. By nurturing and balancing Agni, individuals can foster a vibrant state of health, prevent disease, and promote longevity and well-being. Understanding and respecting the role of Agni is pivotal for anyone seeking to live in alignment with Ayurvedic principles and enjoy a balanced, harmonious life.

1.5 Importance of Ojas, Tejas, and Prana

In Ayurveda, Ojas, Tejas, and Prana are considered the subtle essences that form the foundation of immunity, vitality, intelligence, and life force. These vital energies are interrelated and play a crucial role in maintaining overall health and well-being. Recognizing their importance is essential to harnessing the full potential of Ayurvedic wisdom.

Ojas: The Essence of Vitality and Immunity

- Definition: Ojas is the refined essence of the body's metabolic processes, representing the ultimate nectar of digestion and the fundamental energy reserve. It is associated with immunity, longevity, and physical strength.

- Role in Health: Ojas is responsible for vitality, vigour, and overall immunity. It stabilizes the body and mind, providing strength to endure mental and physical challenges and protecting against illness.

- Signs of Strong Ojas: Individuals with abundant Ojas exhibit radiance, robust health, emotional resilience, and a balanced mind. They experience a deep sense of happiness and spiritual fulfilment.

- Imbalance Symptoms: Diminished Ojas can lead to weakness, fatigue, frequent illness, depression, and emotional instability. It is crucial to nurture Ojas through proper nutrition, rest, spiritual practices, and stress management.

Tejas: The Radiance of Inner Wisdom and Metabolism

- Definition: Tejas is the subtle fire principle, reflecting the transformative aspect of energy, encompassing both metabolism at the cellular level and the illumination of the mind. It emanates from a well-managed Pitta dosha.

- Role in Health: Tejas is essential for digestion, perception, intelligence, and cellular metabolism. It governs clarity of thought, discrimination, and courage.

- Signs of Balanced Tejas: When Tejas is balanced, individuals exhibit intellectual sharpness, perceptive insight, and a vibrant aura. They have a focused, courageous, and self-disciplined nature.

- Imbalance Symptoms: Excess Tejas can manifest as irritability, impatience, excessive heat, and inflammatory conditions. Maintaining Tejas involves cultivating a balanced approach to diet, lifestyle, and stress reduction.

Prana: The Life Force Energy

- Definition: Prana is the vital life force governing the physical and mental actions within the body, akin to the breath of life. It is associated with Vata dosha and is the driving force that animates all functions, from cellular to spiritual.

- Role in Health: Prana facilitates vitality, movement, speech, respiration, and cognition. It allows an individual to interact dynamically with their environment and practice awareness and mindfulness.

- Signs of Adequate Prana: A person with balanced Prana exhibits vitality, alertness, calmness, and creativity. They demonstrate strong communication skills and adaptive, resilient behaviour.

- Imbalance Symptoms: Imbalances in Prana can lead to fatigue, anxiety, shortness of breath, and a scattered mind. Practices such as pranayama (breathing exercises), meditation, and regular physical activity help maintain and balance Prana.

Interconnectedness and Enhancement

Ojas, Tejas, and Prana are interdependent, each influencing and supporting the others:

- Ojas nurtures and stabilizes Prana and Tejas, providing the necessary strength for cognitive and physical activities.
- Tejas refines Prana and Ojas, ensuring there is a balance between transformation and stability.
- Prana energizes Ojas and Tejas, facilitating their functions and enabling adaptability to environmental and internal changes.

To cultivate and maintain these subtle energies, Ayurveda emphasizes a balanced lifestyle that includes nourishing food, disciplined routines, meditation, yoga, and ethical living. These practices promote harmony among Ojas, Tejas, and Prana, contributing to overall health, vitality, spiritual growth, and life's profound richness.

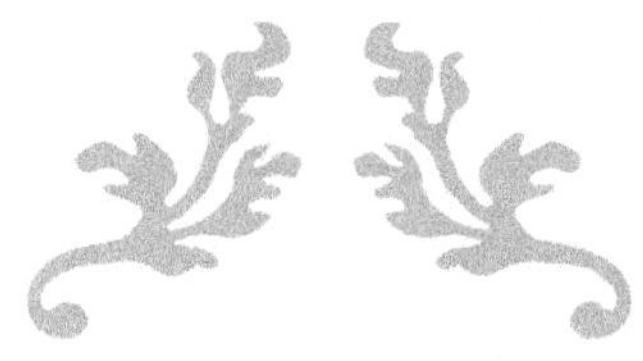

CHAPTER 2 – UNDERSTANDING NADI PARIKSHANA

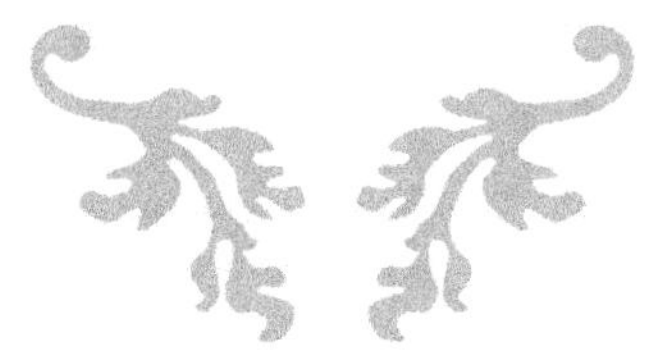

2.1 Historical Perspective and Textual References

Nadi Parikshan, or pulse examination, is an ancient diagnostic practice with deep roots in the Ayurvedic tradition. It has intrigued and guided practitioners for millennia, offering insights into the intricate workings of the human body and mind. Understanding its historical development and textual foundation provides a richer appreciation of its significance and methodology.

Ancient Origins

The origins of Nadi Parikshan can be traced back to the Vedic period, where initial references to pulse examination are found within the sacred texts of Ayurveda. This practice evolved over centuries, earning a revered place among the tools of Ayurvedic diagnosis.

Classical Ayurvedic Texts

1. Charaka Samhita: As one of the foundational texts of Ayurveda, the Charaka Samhita provides detailed descriptions of various diagnostic techniques, including pulse examination. Although it does not elaborate on Nadi Parikshan as extensively as some later texts, it lays the groundwork by emphasizing the importance of understanding the patient's constitution and current imbalances.

2. Sushruta Samhita: This text, attributed to the sage Sushruta, is renowned for its surgical knowledge but also incorporates diagnostic approaches, especially in the context of determining doshic imbalances and dhatu conditions through clinical observation, including pulsation.

3. Ashtanga Hridayam: Compiled by Vagbhata, the Ashtanga Hridayam synthesizes the teachings of earlier Ayurvedic texts and presents a more refined understanding of pulse examination. It discusses the variations in pulse related to doshic changes and is considered pivotal in standardizing the practice.

4. Sharngadhara Samhita: This 14th-century text is particularly significant for its specific focus on Nadi Parikshan. Sharngadhara provides comprehensive insights into the different qualities of the pulse associated with the three doshas and offers detailed methodologies for using pulse examination to diagnose various conditions.

Nadi Parikshan, or pulse diagnosis, has a rich history in Ayurvedic literature, underscoring its significance as a diagnostic tool deeply intertwined with the understanding of the tridoshas—Vata, Pitta, and Kapha. The textual evidence provided in key Ayurvedic texts illustrates the evolution and enduring importance of this practice throughout the centuries.

Key Textual References on Nadi Parikshan

Sharangdhar Samhita (13th Century)

The Sharangdhar Samhita is acknowledged for bringing pulse diagnosis to the forefront in Ayurvedic diagnostics. It was the first text to explicitly identify and articulate the relationship between the pulse (Nadi) and the tridoshas. This marked a pivotal moment in Ayurvedic medicine, as it provided a more systematic approach to diagnosing health states based on the nuances of pulse reading.

Bhavprakash (16th Century)

Written by Shri Bhav Mishra Ji, the Bhavprakash expands upon classical Ayurvedic knowledge and includes references to Nadi Parikshan. This text reinforces the diagnostic role of pulse reading within the broader context of Ayurvedic practice, emphasizing its application in understanding doshic imbalances.

Yogratnakara (17th Century)

The Yogratnakara dedicates a section to the science of Nadi, elaborating on pulse diagnosis in 48 shlokas. This text offers detailed descriptions of pulse qualities and their correlation with health and disease, providing practical guidelines for accurate pulse examination.

Bhela Samhita

An early Ayurvedic text, the Bhela Samhita provides one of the earliest known references to Nadi Pariksha. Its inclusion of pulse diagnosis indicates the long-standing value placed on this method for assessing the internal state of the body.

Harit Samhita

Another foundational work, the Harit Samhita describes Nadi Pariksha as a crucial diagnostic tool, aligning its practice with the assessment of doshic states and contributing to the personalized approach in Ayurveda.

Angivin Nadi Shastra

This early text underscores the role of Nadi Pariksha in Ayurveda, highlighting the connection between the pulse and overall health assessment, which would have informed other texts and practices in traditional medicine.

Bharadwaja Samhita

Attributed to Bharadwaja, this text illustrates the ancient roots of pulse diagnosis, noting its utility in understanding the imbalances within the tridoshas through pulse observation.

Kanada

Kanada's references to Nadi Pariksha further validate the widespread acceptance and application of pulse diagnosis in early Ayurvedic writings, showcasing its importance across different contexts.

Markandeya

The Markandeya text contributes to the traditional knowledge of Nadi Pariksha, adding to the collective wisdom on pulse examination as a tool for determining internal health states.

Ravana

Attributed to the legendary scholar Ravana, this text discusses the relevance of pulse reading in diagnosing doshic imbalances, enhancing the depth of diagnostic methodologies.

Bhudharbhatta

The descriptions provided by Bhudharbhatta contribute to the understanding of Nadi Pariksha, emphasizing its significance in the comprehensive diagnostic frameworks of Ayurveda.

These texts collectively highlight the historical importance and development of Nadi Parikshan as a diagnostic practice. Over centuries, pulse diagnosis has remained integral to Ayurveda, guiding practitioners in the nuanced interpretation of the body's energies for personalized health insights. This enduring tradition underscores the sophistication of ancient diagnostic techniques and their continued relevance in achieving holistic well-being.

Nadi Parikshan Through the Ages

Over the centuries, Ayurvedic practitioners have expanded and refined the knowledge of Nadi Parikshan, drawing upon both textual sources and empirical experience. The practice became more sophisticated, with detailed guidance on the interpretation of pulse qualities based on location, rhythm, speed, and temperature.

While traditional pulse diagnosis relied heavily on empirical wisdom passed down orally from gurus to disciples, its principles and techniques have been preserved and modernized over time, making it accessible to contemporary practitioners.

Integration with Complementary Disciplines

Beyond the primary Ayurvedic texts, references to pulse examination can be found in various Siddha and Unani medicinal scripts, highlighting the cross-cultural and interdisciplinary recognition of its utility in health assessment and personalized medicine.

Nadi Parikshan's rich history and enduring presence in Ayurvedic texts underscore its value as a diagnostic tool. By grounding our understanding in its historical context and classical references, we continue to honour and advance this profound practice. This historical perspective not only reminds us of the deep wisdom embedded in Ayurvedic traditions but also propels us to integrate such knowledge with contemporary health paradigms, ensuring its relevance and application for future generations.

<u>2.2 Methodology of Nadi Pariksha</u>

Nadi Pariksha, or pulse diagnosis, is a sophisticated and nuanced assessment method that involves interpreting the subtle qualities of the pulse to gain insights into an individual's health. It is a cornerstone of Ayurvedic diagnosis, offering a window into the balance (or imbalance) of the tridoshas—Vata, Pitta, and Kapha—and providing guidance for personalized treatment plans. The methodology of Nadi Pariksha is an art and science that requires sensitivity, intuition, and experience.

Preparation and Environment

- Practitioner Readiness: Before performing Nadi Pariksha, the practitioner should be in a calm and centered state of mind, free from distractions, to enhance sensitivity and receptivity.
- Setting: The examination should be conducted in a quiet and comfortable environment. The patient should be relaxed and seated comfortably, with their arm supported at heart level to avoid tension or strain.

The Process of Pulse Examination

1. Positioning the Hand:

  - The patient is asked to extend their left arm (for females) or right arm (for males). This preference is rooted in traditional beliefs but can be adapted based on the practitioner's discretion.
  - The arm is slightly bent, with the palm facing upward. The elbow should rest comfortably on a table or the practitioner's arm to ensure stability.

2. Placement of Fingers:

- The practitioner uses the index, middle, and ring fingers of their dominant hand to assess the pulse.

- The fingers are placed gently on the radial artery at the wrist, just above the base of the thumb. Each finger's placement corresponds to sensing one of the three doshas:
  - Index finger for Vata
  - Middle finger for Pitta
  - Ring finger for Kapha

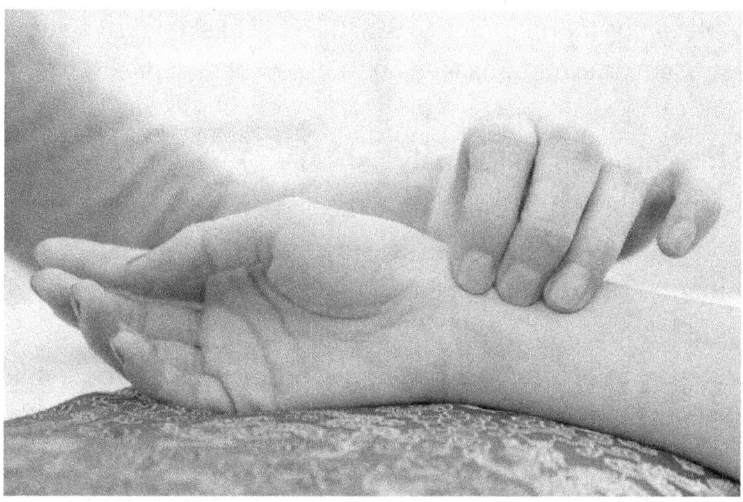

3. Assessing the Pulse:

- Depth and Pressure: The practitioner applies light, moderate, and deep pressure with their fingers to assess the pulse at different levels, providing insights into superficial and deep-seated imbalances.

- Rate and Rhythm: The pulse's rate (beats per minute) and rhythm (regularity and sprint) give clues about the overall state of the doshas.

- Qualities of the Pulse: Traditional Ayurveda describes specific pulse qualities associated with each dosha:

- Vata Pulse: Light, thin, and irregular like a snake.
- Pitta Pulse: Sharp, intense, and bounding like a frog.
- Kapha Pulse: Slow, steady, and strong like a swan.

4. Interpreting Variations:

- Combinations of doshic pulses may be felt, indicating complex imbalances or specific health conditions.
- The practitioner considers other qualities and nuances such as temperature, volume, tension, and consistency of the pulse, integrating this information with the patient's medical history and presenting symptoms for a holistic view of their health.

Interpretation and Analysis

- Correlation with Symptoms: The findings from Nadi Pariksha are compared with the patient's symptoms, lifestyle, and Prakriti (constitution) to formulate a comprehensive health assessment.
- Identifying Imbalances: By recognizing the dominance or deficiency of the doshas, practitioners can pinpoint potential health issues or predispositions, guiding relevant therapeutic interventions.
- Monitoring Progress: Nadi Pariksha serves as an ongoing diagnostic tool to monitor the patient's response to treatments and adjust care plans accordingly.

The methodology of Nadi Pariksha is both an art and a science, necessitating years of experience and intuitive understanding. It offers invaluable diagnostic insights, transcending physical symptoms to evaluate broader physiological and psychological states. This timeless practice is indispensable in providing personalized care, underlining Ayurveda's emphasis on treating the individual as a whole.

2.3 Tools and Techniques Used

Nadi Pariksha, despite its ancient origins, primarily relies on the practitioner's skill and sensitivity rather than on sophisticated instruments. However, there are essential tools and techniques involved that enhance the efficiency and accuracy of this practice. The emphasis in pulse diagnosis is on developing acute perceptual abilities and understanding the qualitative nuances of the pulse.

Tools Used in Nadi Pariksha

1. Practitioner's Fingers:

 - The primary tool in Nadi Pariksha is the practitioner's own fingers, particularly the index, middle, and ring fingers of the dominant hand. These are used to feel the pulse at varying depths and pressures, allowing the practitioner to discern the qualities associated with each of the three doshas.

2. Comfortable Examination Setting:

 - A sturdy chair and table or a cushioned surface that supports the patient's arm are essential to ensure comfort and stability during the examination, allowing both patient and practitioner to focus on the subtle nuances of the pulse.

3. Chronometer or Watch:

 - While traditional practitioners rely on intuition and experience to count the pulse rate, a watch or chronometer can be used to accurately determine the pulse rate and rhythm per minute, especially valuable for less experienced practitioners or for documentation purposes.

4. Notebook or Recording Device:
   - A notebook or digital device is useful for recording observations, findings, and treatment recommendations. Documenting pulse characteristics over time can help track the patient's progress and response to treatment.

Techniques Used in Nadi Pariksha

1. Finger Placement and Pressure:
   - Placement: The practitioner places their fingers lightly on the radial artery of the patient's wrist, using the different fingers to correspond to the doshas (index for Vata, middle for Pitta, and ring for Kapha).
   - Pressure Levels: Applying light, moderate, and deep pressure allows the practitioner to assess superficial and deep characteristics of the pulse, providing a comprehensive view of the patient's health.

2. Pulse Quality Assessment:
   - The practitioner assesses various pulse qualities, including:
   - Rate: Counting the number of beats per minute gives insight into the metabolic and energetic state of the patient.
   - Rhythm: Evaluating the regularity and rhythm helps in understanding the balance or imbalance within the doshas.
   - Force and Volume: Noting the strength of the pulse and any variations in force can indicate the health of specific organs or systems.
   - Temperature: Attention to the warmth or coolness of the pulse site can provide additional diagnostic information.

3. Visualization Techniques:

- Experienced practitioners often use visualization techniques to enhance their sensitivity and focus during pulse examination, imagining the flow of energy or picturing the qualities of each dosha.

4. Corroborative Techniques:
  - Pulse diagnosis is often used in conjunction with other diagnostic methods such as clinical observation, enquiry about the patient's lifestyle and symptoms, and examination of the tongue, eyes, and other physical features to build a holistic assessment.

5. Integrated Analysis:
  - The practitioner synthesizes the findings from the pulse examination with knowledge of the patient's medical history, constitution, and current symptoms to devise a personalized treatment plan.

While the tools used in Nadi Pariksha may be simple, the techniques require meticulous practice, sharp intuition, and an in-depth understanding of Ayurvedic principles. Mastery of these techniques allows practitioners to harness the full potential of pulse diagnosis, providing insights into the intricate balance of the tridoshas and fostering a deep understanding of the individual's health and well-being.

Additional Tools for Nadi Pariksha

1. Pulse Chart/Guide:
  - Visual aids or charts that outline the characteristics of Vata, Pitta, and Kapha pulses can be valuable educational tools for students and novice practitioners, helping them to identify and memorize the subtle nuances of each dosha.

2. Pulse Oximeter:

- While not traditionally part of Ayurveda, a pulse oximeter can be used to measure heart rate and oxygen saturation, providing supplemental data that can be aligned with subjective pulse assessment findings.

3. Digital Pulse Diagnostic Devices:

- Emerging technology includes digital pulse diagnostic tools that analyse pulse data in detail. These devices measure and interpret various parameters such as rhythm, elasticity, and volume, offering additional insights alongside traditional assessment.

- Such tools can be especially useful in teaching settings or for practitioners who wish to verify and correlate their findings with objective data.

4. Temperature Sensors:

- Infrared thermometers or contact temperature sensors can measure the temperature at the pulse site, aiding in the assessment of Pitta imbalances or inflammatory conditions.

5. Biofeedback Tools:

- Biofeedback devices can assist in monitoring physiological parameters like heart rate variability, which may provide deeper insights into the autonomic nervous system's response to stress and relaxation, complementing pulse diagnosis.

6. Stethoscope:

- Though not commonly associated with Ayurveda, a stethoscope may be used to cross-reference findings by listening to heart sounds, aiding in a more comprehensive cardiovascular assessment.

7. Feedback and Learning Systems:

   - Software programs or apps designed for Ayurvedic learning can simulate pulse examination scenarios, providing interactive platforms for practitioners to practice and refine their pulse reading skills.

8. Collaborative Diagnostic Platforms:

   - Platforms that allow for sharing of pulse data with other practitioners or specialists can foster collaborative diagnosis, providing multiple perspectives that may enhance the understanding of complex health conditions.

While the essence of Nadi Pariksha remains the practitioner's ability to sense and interpret the pulse manually, these additional tools can complement traditional techniques, offer educational support, and foster integration with modern diagnostic practices. The key is to use these tools as complements to the inherent wisdom of Ayurveda, ensuring they serve to enrich the practitioner's insights rather than replace the subtle art and intuition integral to pulse diagnosis.

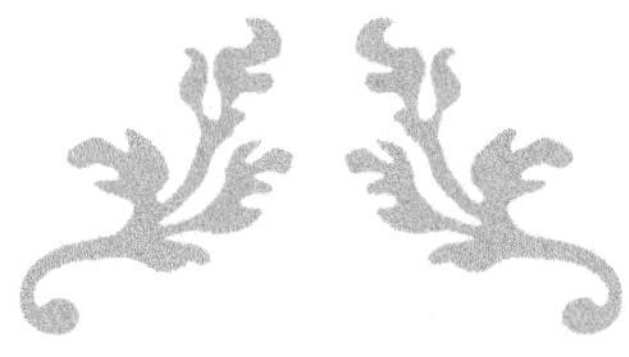

CHAPTER 3 – PHYSIOLOGY OF PULSE IN AYURVEDA

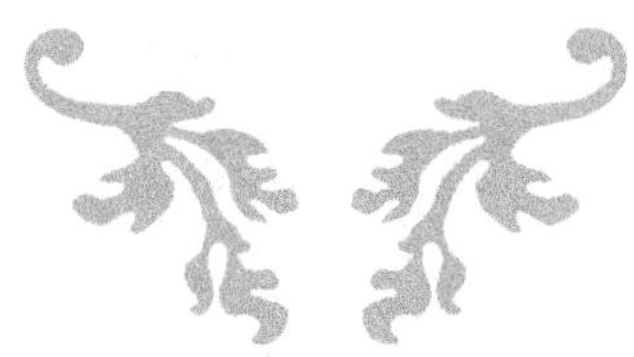

3.1 Characteristics of Vata Pulse

In Ayurveda, the characteristics of the Vata pulse are intricately linked to the elemental qualities of air and space, which define this dosha. Vata, being the force of movement and communication, imparts certain distinctive features to the pulse. Understanding these characteristics is essential for practitioners of Nadi Parikshan (pulse diagnosis) to accurately assess the underlying physiological processes governed by Vata in an individual.

1. Quality of Movement

The Vata pulse is primarily characterized by its movement. It is often described using analogies that capture its unique qualities:
- Snake-like (Sarpa Gati): The Vata pulse moves in a serpentine manner, with a subtle, undulating motion. This characteristic reflects the agile and erratic nature of Vata, which embodies the movement and flow within the body.

2. Speed and Rhythm

The Vata pulse exhibits distinct speed and rhythm qualities:
- Fast Pace: The pulse of Vata displays a rapid pace. It beats swiftly, often perceived as faster than the pulsations associated with the other doshas.
- Irregular Rhythm: There is an irregularity in the rhythm of a Vata pulse, mirroring the unpredictable and variable nature of this dosha. It may skip beats or alter its rhythm spontaneously.

3. Pressure and Depth

The tactile sensation of the Vata pulse is defined by:

- Light Pressure: When feeling the Vata pulse, practitioners note its lightness. It exerts a gentle pressure against the fingertips, as if dancing just beneath the skin.
- Superficial Depth: The Vata pulse is typically closer to the surface, floating near the skin, indicative of its less tangible, airy qualities.

4. Temperature and Volume

These additional characteristics help refine the understanding of the Vata pulse:
- Cool Temperature: The Vata pulse may feel cooler to the touch, reflecting the coolness attributed to the air element.
- Low Volume: The volume of the Vata pulse is often subdued, presenting as a weak or thready beat, consistent with the lighter, more subtle energy of Vata.

5. Texture

Texture further differentiates the Vata pulse:
- Dryness: There is a perceived dryness in the quality of the Vata pulse. It lacks the moisture or oiliness seen in pulses dominated by other elements.
- Roughness: The pulse may convey a sense of roughness or a less smooth texture, resonating with the dry and rough qualities inherent in Vata.

6. Variability

One of the most defining attributes of the Vata pulse is its variability:
- Unpredictability: The Vata pulse is prone to changeability. Its speed, depth, and rhythm can alter quickly and unexpectedly, echoing Vata's dynamic and mutable tendencies.

7. Thready and Fine

The Vata pulse is often described in terms of its size and feel:

- Thready Pulse: It can appear thin and thready, almost like a thin string beneath the fingertips. This description aligns with the inherent lightness and subtlety of Vata.
- Fine Quality: The pulse exudes a fine, delicate sensation, again reflective of the ethereal nature of the air and space it embodies.

8. Contractions and Expansions

The Vata pulse may exhibit a unique pattern of movement:

- Frequent Contractions: This pulse can palpably exhibit frequent contractions, moments of tighter rhythmic interaction, followed by periods of relaxation.
- Sudden Expansions: These contractions may be interspersed with sudden expansions, providing a distinct pulsatile nature that is not easily predicted.

The Vata pulse is a fascinating indicator of the dynamic and ever-changing energies at play within the body. Its snake-like movement, rapid and irregular rhythm, light and superficial presence, cool temperature, and variability are signature features that practitioners learn to recognize through skillful practice. Understanding these nuances allows Ayurvedic practitioners to assess how well Vata is balanced within an individual, thereby guiding personalized approaches to nurture coherence and health. Each characteristic, felt through careful palpation and perceptive insight, deepens the practitioner's connection to the body's subtle communications and the holistic vision of Ayurveda.

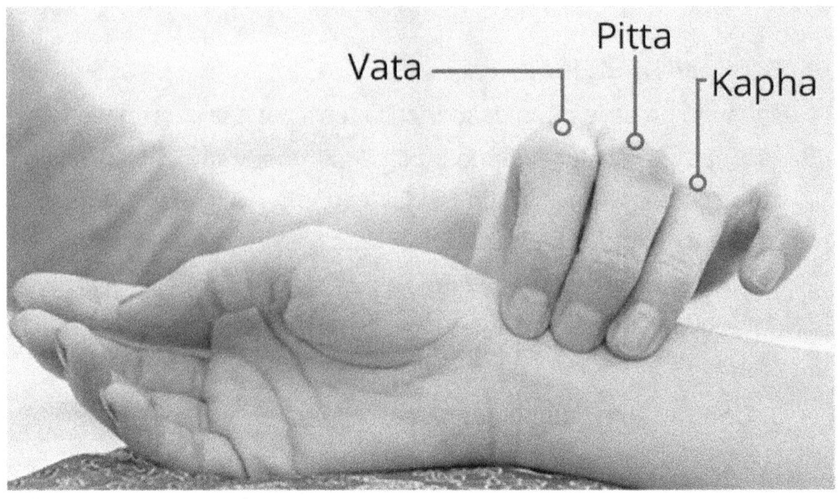

3.2 Characteristics of Pitta Pulse

The Pitta pulse, governed by the fire and water elements, reflects the transformative and metabolic nature of this dosha. It embodies the qualities of heat, sharpness, and intensity, mirroring the roles Pitta plays in digestion, metabolism, and intellectual processes. Ayurvedic practitioners trained in Nadi Parikshan (pulse diagnosis) develop an understanding of these characteristics to assess the balance of Pitta within an individual.

1. Quality of Movement

The Pitta pulse exhibits a distinct quality of movement:

- Frog-like (Manduca Gati): Often described as frog-like, the Pitta pulse has a jumping or bounding characteristic. This portrayal captures the energetic and purposeful movement inherent to Pitta.

2. Speed and Rhythm

Pitta's energetic nature is reflected in its speed and rhythm:

- Moderate to Fast Pace: The Pitta pulse beats at a moderate to fast pace, reflecting the active metabolic processes governed by the Pitta dosha.

- Steady Rhythm: Unlike the irregular pattern of Vata, the Pitta pulse maintains a more regular and predictable rhythm, signifying an organized and intentional energy flow.

3. Pressure and Depth

The sensation of the pulse beneath the fingers is significantly influenced by Pitta:

- Moderate Pressure: The Pitta pulse exerts a moderate pressure, creating a sense of firmness and clarity as it is felt by the practitioner.

- Mid-Level Depth: It typically resides at a moderate depth, neither too superficial nor too deep, indicating Pitta's balanced precipitation between form and energy.

4. Temperature and Volume

The heat of Pitta manifests in its temperature and volume:

- Warm Temperature: A distinctive feature of the Pitta pulse is its warmth, a direct expression of the fire element predominant in this dosha.

- Strong Volume: The pulse often feels full-bodied and robust, indicative of the intensity and vigour associated with Pitta.

5. Texture

Texture provides additional insight into the Pitta pulse:

- Oily Texture: The feel of the Pitta pulse can be smooth and somewhat oily, reflecting the fluid component of Pitta's fire and water elements.
- Sharpness: There is a palpable sharpness to the pulse, echoing the penetrating and focused nature of Pitta.

6. Consistency and Regularity

These features mark the distinctive consistency of the Pitta pulse:
- Consistent: The Pitta pulse is consistently felt throughout the examination, reliable in its beats, resonating with the organized and systematic nature of Pitta's heat-driven processes.
- Predictable: Predictability is key, with a rhythm that aligns with the methodical action of this dosha.

7. Vibrant and Forceful

The Pitta pulse communicates vitality and strength:
- Vibrant Pulse: Its vibrant quality implies lively metabolic activities, a hallmark of healthy and active Pitta.
- Forceful: There is a forcefulness to the pulse, signifying strong digestive and assimilative capabilities crucial for maintaining health.

8. Expansive and Attentive

These attributes speak to Pitta's dynamic energy:
- Expansive Nature: The pulse can occasionally expand intensely, reflecting the transformative energy and dynamism of Pitta.
- Attentive Pulse: The Pitta pulse displays a focused alertness, paralleling the clarity and discriminative abilities governed by this dosha.

The Pitta pulse is an embodiment of the transformative and metabolic energies central to human physiology. Its frog-like movement, moderate to fast pace, steady rhythm, warm and strong presence, and oily yet sharp texture are hallmarks that Ayurvedic practitioners learn to interpret through diligent practice and sensitivity. Recognizing these characteristics allows for an insightful assessment of how Pitta influences an individual's physiological and psychological states, guiding personalized recommendations to maintain balance. Therefore, the characteristics of the Pitta pulse not only represent the fiery nature of this dosha but also serve as a touchstone for comprehending the body's resourceful and transformative capacities within the deep tradition of Ayurveda.

3.3 Characteristics of Kapha Pulse

The Kapha pulse represents the qualities of stability, structure, and cohesion, rooted in the water and earth elements that define this dosha. Kapha's influence in the body is synonymous with growth, strength, and endurance, and its pulse characteristics reflect these essential roles. Mastering the identification and interpretation of the Kapha pulse through Nadi Pariksha (pulse diagnosis) is a critical skill for Ayurvedic practitioners, allowing them to evaluate the body's state of balance and groundedness.

1. Quality of Movement
The movement quality of the Kapha pulse is distinct:
- Swan-like (Hamsa Gati): The Kapha pulse is often likened to the smooth, graceful movement of a swan. This imagery reflects the slow, steady, and deliberate nature of Kapha, emphasizing its stabilizing and grounding properties.

2. Speed and Rhythm

In contrast to the other doshas, Kapha's speed and rhythm are characterized by:

- Slow Pace: The pulse beats with a slower pace, indicative of the steady, enduring quality of Kapha.
- Regular Rhythm: The rhythm is consistent and predictable, mirroring Kapha's methodical and reliable attributes.

3. Pressure and Depth

The sensation of the pulse in terms of pressure and depth reveals much about Kapha:
- Heavy Pressure: The Kapha pulse exerts a firm and heavy pressure, symbolizing its density and strength.
- Deep Depth: It is typically felt at a deeper level, aligning with Kapha's association with foundational strength and support within the body.

4. Temperature and Volume

Kapha's stabilizing influence is evident in its temperature and volume:
- Cool Temperature: The pulse often feels cool to the touch, resonating with the cool, moist nature of the dosha.
- Full Volume: It has a large, full-bodied presence, affirming Kapha's physical robustness and its role in nutrient storage and structural integrity.

5. Texture

The texture of the Kapha pulse is informing:

- Smooth Texture: The pulse is smooth and flowing, reflecting the oily and slippery qualities attributed to the moisture content in Kapha.

- Solid: There is a palpably solid feel to the pulse, consistent with the earthiness that underpins Kapha's manifestations.

6. Consistency and Solidity

Consistency characterizes the Kapha pulse:

- Uniform Consistency: The pulse maintains a uniform quality, unfaltering and dependable over time, mirroring the consistency and stability Kapha provides.

- Solid Beat: The beat of the Kapha pulse is robust and secure, emphasizing strength and stability.

7. Grounded and Anchoring

The Kapha pulse inherently possesses grounding properties:

- Grounded Pulse: Its grounded nature signifies the foundational support Kapha offers in both physical and emotional stability.

- Anchoring: The pulse acts as an anchor, providing a sense of rootedness and security, important for maintaining balance and harmony.

8. Deeply Resonant

Resonance is a significant characteristic of the Kapha pulse:

- Resonant Quality: The pulse's resonant quality contributes to its echoing presence, symbolizing the internal reverberation of Kapha's cohesive energy.

- Echoing Stability: This echoing effect signals stability, akin to a constant, reverberating cadence within the body's systems.

The Kapha pulse is a manifestation of the stabilizing, nurturing, and cohesive energies essential to maintaining health and structural integrity. Its swan-like movement, slow pace, regular rhythm, heavy and deep presence, cool temperature, and groundedness are all characteristics that Ayurvedic practitioners learn to discern through attentive practice. By understanding and interpreting the Kapha pulse, practitioners can assess how well this dosha is supporting an individual's physiological and psychological equilibrium, guiding informed strategies to sustain or restore balance. These characteristics illustrate the nurturing and protective nature of Kapha, which plays a vital role in the holistic understanding of health within the Ayurvedic framework.

3.4 Understanding Combination Pulses

In Ayurveda, combination pulses represent the dynamic interplay between the doshas—Vata, Pitta, and Kapha—reflecting the complex and unique constitution of each individual. These pulses offer a comprehensive insight into how various doshic energies manifest in unison, often indicating a nuanced balance or imbalance that requires careful assessment by the practitioner.

Combination pulses arise when two or more of the doshas express their qualities simultaneously or in succession within the pulse. Understanding these combinations is crucial for accurate diagnosis and personalized treatment planning in Ayurvedic practice.

1. Vata-Pitta Pulse

The Vata-Pitta pulse showcases characteristics indicative of both movement and metabolism:

- Characteristics:

- Movement and Speed: The pulse has a swift pace, characteristic of Vata, combined with a noticeable steadiness or regularity from Pitta.
- Irregular Yet Sharp: It might exhibit irregularity from Vata, yet with a sharpness contributed by Pitta.
- Warm and Light Pressure: The pulse temperature can be warm, a Pitta trait, with a light pressure typical of Vata.

- Interpretation:
- Practitioners may recognize the quick yet penetrating nature of this pulse, often indicating heightening energetic activity in the body, such as metabolism and nervous system function, necessitating attention to balance both stimulation and digestion.

2. Vata-Kapha Pulse

A Vata-Kapha pulse embodies characteristics of movement and stability:
- Characteristics:
- Rhythm and Depth: The pulse is likely to be slow and steady, a Kapha hallmark, yet with the unpredictable rhythm typical of Vata.
- Cool and Light: It may feel cool, pointing to Kapha, while retaining a light pressure attribute from Vata.
- Superficial and Heavy: Exhibits variability in depth, being both superficial like Vata and heavier in presence like Kapha.

- Interpretation:
- This combination suggests a dynamic between mobility and structural cohesion, often requiring interventions that align with grounding practices for Vata and energizing strategies for Kapha to harmonize movement and retention in the body.

3. Pitta-Kapha Pulse

The Pitta-Kapha pulse blends the transformative and stabilizing qualities:

- Characteristics:

  - Force and Consistency: Strong and consistent force typical of Kapha, with underlying intensity indicative of Pitta.

  - Warm and Oily: Exhibits a warm temperature from Pitta and an oily texture due to Kapha.

  - Firm and Regular: A firm beat reflecting Kapha's solid characteristics, alongside Pitta's consistent rhythm.

- Interpretation:

  - A Pitta-Kapha pulse points to intense metabolic functions with solid stability, suggesting potential inflammatory processes accompanied by fluid retention, directing towards strategies that moderate heat and maintain fluid balance.

4. Tridoshic Pulse (Vata-Pitta-Kapha)

The Tridoshic pulse is characterized by the presence of qualities from all three doshas:

- Characteristics:

  - Diverse Qualities: This pulse exhibits qualities that shift between light, sharp, and heavy pressures, encapsulating the distinctive attributes of Vata, Pitta, and Kapha.

  - Warm, Cool, and Balanced Temperature: Temperatures may fluctuate, presenting warmth, coolness, or moderation.

  - Adaptable Rhythm and Depth: A varying rhythm and depth, alternately reflecting mobility, sharpness, and stability.

- Interpretation:

- The Tridoshic pulse often signals a balanced state or, conversely, a complex imbalance that impacts the whole system. Diagnosis and treatment necessitate comprehensive strategies that address all doshas, reinforcing foundational balance and personalized dietary and lifestyle adjustments.

Combination pulses in Ayurveda provide a profound understanding of an individual's doshic dynamics and are pivotal in crafting tailored therapeutic interventions. By grasping the subtleties of combination pulses, practitioners can more accurately decipher how the doshas interact, highlighting potential areas for intervention or support. These insights into the body's energetic harmonies and tensions enable a holistic approach to health, forming the basis for personalized, effective Ayurvedic care.

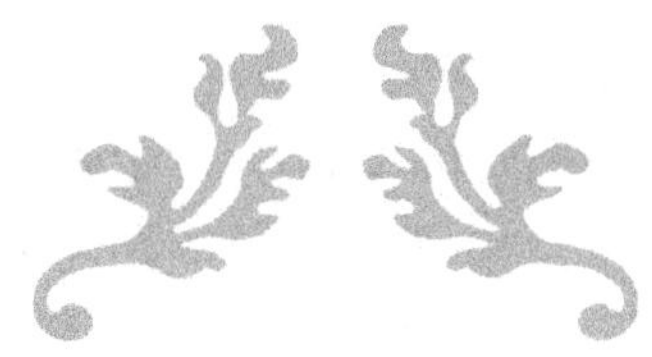

CHAPTER 4 –
DIAGNOSTIC
INSIGHTS FROM
NADI PARIKSHAN

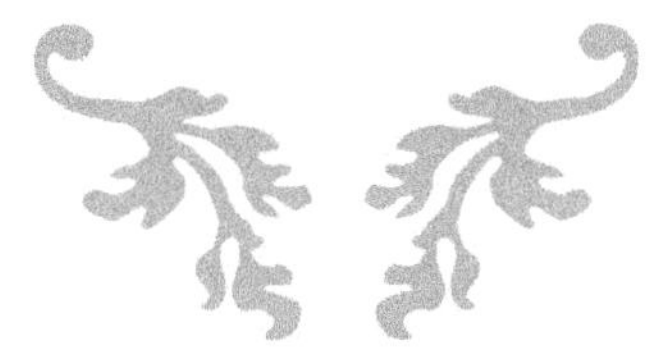

4.1 Dosha Imbalances and Their Pulse Manifestations

In Ayurveda, understanding dosha imbalances is crucial for diagnosing health conditions and implementing effective treatment strategies. These imbalances—known as "Vikriti"—manifest noticeably in the pulse, allowing skilled practitioners to discern underlying health issues. Through Nadi Parikshan (pulse diagnosis), practitioners analyse the pulse's specific qualities, seeking insights into which dosha is in excess or deficiency and how these imbalances impact the body and mind.

Below we explore how each dosha's imbalance can reflect in pulse characteristics:

Vata Imbalance

When Vata is imbalanced, its pulse manifestations often reflect its aggravated qualities of coldness, dryness, and irregular movement:

- Characteristics of Vata-Imbalanced Pulse:
  - Increased Irregularity: The pulse becomes more erratic, with an unpredictable rhythm and frequent skips.
  - Rapid Changes: Quick or abrupt changes in rate and quality, showcasing heightened variability.
  - Light and Weak: The pulse is lighter and weaker, possibly thready, signifying Vata's intoxication of movement and dispersion.
  - Cool and Rough Texture: Feel cooler to the touch, with a potential roughness or lack of smoothness seen in their texture.

- Indicative Symptoms:
   - Anxiety, insomnia, restlessness, cold extremities, dry skin, and irregular digestion, are often linked with an imbalanced Vata.

Pitta Imbalance

Pitta imbalances bring about increased heat and intensity, which is mirrored in pulse manifestations:

- Characteristics of Pitta-Imbalanced Pulse:
   - Sharp and Forceful: Pulse feels sharp and forceful, indicative of heightened intensity and heat.
   - Rapid and Strong Rhythm: Demonstrates a fast, persistent rhythm, with forceful throbbing.
   - Warm Temperature: The pulse is often warm or hot to the touch, resonating with Pitta's fiery nature.
   - Oily Texture: There may be a slight oily or greasy quality to the pulse, reflective of Pitta's lubrication.

- Indicative Symptoms:
   - Inflammatory conditions, heartburn, skin rashes, excessive hunger or thirst, and irritability often accompany Pitta imbalances.

Kapha Imbalance

Kapha imbalances, characterized by stagnation, heaviness, and coolness, are reflected in distinctive pulse features:

- Characteristics of Kapha-Imbalanced Pulse:
   - Sluggish and Heavy: The pulse displays a sluggish and heavy quality, often presenting as excessively full.

- Slow and Stable Rhythm: The rhythm is slow and steady but lacks vibrancy or vigour.
- Cool and Moist Texture: Cool to the touch with a moist, slippery texture indicative of Kapha's water element.
- Lack of Clarity: Pulse may feel dull or lacking in distinctness, mirroring Kapha's cloudiness and congestion.

- Indicative Symptoms:
- Lethargy, congestion, weight gain, fluid retention, and depressive states are manifestations of a Kapha imbalance.

Mastering Pulse Diagnosis for Dosha Imbalances

Accurately interpreting these pulse manifestations requires experience and to make aware or responsive to the subtle nuances of Nadi Parikshan. Practitioners consider the qualitative sensations they perceive with their fingertips, drawing on their understanding of Ayurveda's principles to correlate these sensations with potential health conditions.

In practice, recognizing dosha imbalances through pulse assessment allows Ayurvedic practitioners to:

- Tailor Treatments: Customized treatment plans that restore balance, including dietary changes, lifestyle modifications, herbal therapies, and yoga practices.
- Prevent Disease: Identify imbalances before they manifest as more severe health conditions, allowing for preventative interventions.
- Monitor Progress: Utilize pulse characteristics to gauge the effectiveness of treatments and make necessary adjustments.

Understanding the manifestation of dosha imbalances in the pulse is an invaluable skill in Ayurvedic diagnosis. These manifestations act as a diagnostic compass, guiding practitioners toward comprehending the complex interplay of bodily functions and energetic dynamics. By tuning into the pulse's language of imbalance, Ayurveda practitioners contribute to holistic well-being, crafting individualized care paths that realign body, mind, and spirit.

4.2 Identifying Dhatu (Tissue) and Mala (Waste) Conditions

In Ayurveda, health and disease are understood through the framework of the doshas, dhatus (tissues), and malas (wastes). The dhatus are the fundamental bodily tissues, while malas are the waste products that result from metabolic processes. An imbalance or dysfunction in these components can lead to various health issues. Through Nadi Parikshan (pulse diagnosis), practitioners can assess the state of the dhatus and malas, providing insight into a person's overall health and identifying potential areas of concern.

Assessing Dhatu Conditions

The dhatus are sequentially formed from the essence of the digested food, each layer providing nourishment and support to the next. There are seven primary dhatus:

1. Rasa (Plasma/Lymph):
   - Pulse Indicator: A weak, feeble pulse may indicate low Rasa, possibly due to dehydration or poor nutrient absorption.

- Symptoms: Fatigue, poor circulation, lack of vitality, and dehydration.

2. Rakta (Blood):
   - Pulse Indicator: A rapid, forceful pulse can signify excess Rakta, often associated with Pitta imbalances.
   - Symptoms: Skin conditions, inflammation, hypertension, and a tendency toward bleeding.

3. Mamsa (Muscle):
   - Pulse Indicator: A heavy and slow pulse might suggest Mamsa imbalance, typically related to Kapha conditions.
   - Symptoms: Muscular rigidity, heaviness, and obesity.

4. Meda (Fat):
   - Pulse Indicator: A soft, yielding pulse can indicate an imbalance in Meda, often linked with excessive Kapha.
   - Symptoms: Weight gain, high cholesterol, and lethargy.

5. Asthi (Bone):
   - Pulse Indicator: A rough, irregular pulse may reflect Asthi issues, often resulting from Vata imbalances.
   - Symptoms: Joint pain, osteoporosis, and brittleness of nails and hair.

6. Majja (Marrow/Nervous Tissue):
   - Pulse Indicator: A deep, sluggish pulse can indicate Majja imbalances, often tied to Kapha or Vata disturbances.
   - Symptoms: Nervous exhaustion, cognitive issues, and weakness.

7. Shukra (Reproductive Tissue):
  - Pulse Indicator: An oscillating, subtle pulse might reveal Shukra imbalances, particularly when Vata is involved.
  - Symptoms: Infertility, low libido, and reproductive health issues.

Assessing Mala Conditions

The malas are the waste products eliminated from the body, including urine, faeces, and sweat. Proper elimination is crucial for maintaining health, and imbalances can manifest in the pulse:

1. Purisha (Faeces):
  - Pulse Indicator: A sluggish, heavy pulse may suggest compromised Purisha elimination, often linked to Kapha dominance.
  - Symptoms: Constipation, bloating, and abdominal discomfort.

2. Mutra (Urine):
  - Pulse Indicator: A tense, bounding pulse could indicate Mutra imbalance, such as Pitta-related urinary issues.
  - Symptoms: Burning urination, frequent trips to urinate, and dehydration.

3. Sveda (Sweat):
  - Pulse Indicator: A moist, oily pulse may reflect excessive Sveda, commonly associated with Pitta doshic conditions.
  - Symptoms: Excessive sweating, body odour, and skin rashes.

Integrating Pulse Findings with Other Diagnostic Tools

- Observation and Inquiry: In addition to pulse reading, practitioners corroborate findings through visual observation and patient interviews, assessing symptoms and lifestyle factors impacting the dhatus and malas.

- Holistic Diagnosis: Using the pulse as a key diagnostic tool, practitioners gain a comprehensive view of the individual's health, identifying specific tissue and waste-related challenges that may need attention.

The ability to identify conditions of the dhatus and malas through pulse diagnosis is a testament to the depth and precision of Ayurvedic assessment. By understanding how these tissues and wastes manifest in the pulse, practitioners can craft more nuanced and effective treatment plans. This approach not only addresses current health challenges but also supports the maintenance of balance and vitality, reinforcing Ayurveda's holistic vision of health that encompasses body, mind, and spirit.

4.3 Psychological and Mental State Assessment

In Ayurveda, the mind is considered integral to health, influencing and reflecting the state of the body. Psychological and mental states are closely linked with the balance of doshas, the subtle energies of the mind (sattva, rajas, and tamas), and overall lifestyle. Through Nadi Parikshan (pulse diagnosis), practitioners can gain insight into an individual's psychological and mental well-being, offering a profound understanding of how emotional and mental states influence physical health.

Pulse Characteristics and Mental States

Vata and the Mind

- Pulse Characteristics:
  - A pulsating, irregular, and light pulse may suggest Vata's influence on the mind, aligning with characteristics of movement and change.

- Mental and Psychological Manifestations:
  - Increased Vata can lead to anxiety, restlessness, fear, and overthinking. Creativity and quick thinking are enhanced but may tilt toward nervous energy and difficulty focusing.

Pitta and the Mind

- Pulse Characteristics:
  - A sharp, intense, and moderately fast pulse may indicate heightened Pitta, associated with focus and transformation.

- Mental and Psychological Manifestations:
  - When Pitta is elevated, it can lead to irritability, anger, and overly critical thinking. Pitta provides clarity and decisiveness but can result in burnout and aggression if unbalanced.

Kapha and the Mind

- Pulse Characteristics:
  - A slow, steady, and heavy pulse might reflect Kapha's impact on mental states, contributing to calmness and stability.

- Mental and Psychological Manifestations:
  - Excessive Kapha can lead to lethargy, depression, attachment, and resistance to change. Kapha supports resilience and patience but can cause sluggish thinking and emotional withdrawal.

Subtle Energies and Mental Health

Beyond doshas, the subtle energies—sattva, rajas, and tamas—play a vital role in mental health:

- Sattva (Clarity and Purity):
  - Promotes wisdom, compassion, and mental harmony. A balance of sattva leads to clarity of thought, emotional balance, and a tendency toward spiritual growth.

- Rajas (Activity and Change):
  - Associated with action, passion, and excitement. An excess of rajas results in restlessness, desire, and distraction, disrupting mental peace.

- Tamas (Inertia and Darkness):
  - Leads to heaviness, confusion, and apathy. When dominant, tamas may manifest as depression, ignorance, and lack of motivation.

Assessment and Integration with Other Diagnostic Tools

- Pulse as a Mirror:
  - The pulse serves as a mirror of mental states, revealing how thoughts and emotions interplay with physical health. Practitioners interpret pulse qualities in the context of the individual's overall lifestyle, stressors, and emotional resilience.

- Holistic Inquiry:
  - Through dialogue, practitioners further explore the individual's mental and emotional experiences, correlating these insights with pulse findings to develop a coherent picture of mental health.

Crafting a Personalized Approach

The information garnered from pulse diagnosis enables practitioners to craft personalized interventions that address both mental and physical health. This may involve:

- Dietary and Lifestyle Adjustments:
  - Specific foods, routines, and activities can promote mental balance, enhancing sattva and reducing excess rajas or tamas.

- Herbal Remedies:
  - Ayurvedic herbs like Brahmi, Ashwagandha, and Shankhapushpi can support mental clarity, reduce anxiety, and combat depression.

- Mind-Body Practices:
  - Techniques such as meditation, yoga, and pranayama foster mental equilibrium, aligning the subtle energies with the individual's unique constitution.

- Psychological Support:
  - Encouraging self-reflection, emotional expression, and supportive relationships are crucial for sustaining long-term mental well-being.

Nadi Parikshan offers a comprehensive lens through which practitioners can assess psychological and mental states, embodying Ayurveda's holistic approach to health. By understanding the interconnectedness of mind and body, Ayurvedic practitioners help individuals cultivate a balanced mental state, promoting well-being and resilience across life's challenges. This integrative perspective underscores the richness

of Ayurvedic wisdom in nurturing comprehensive health,
addressing the entire spectrum of human experience.

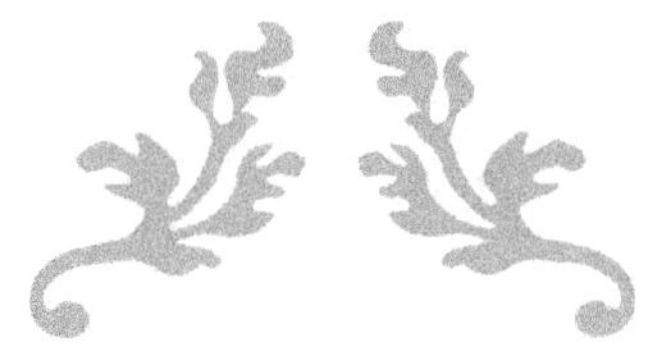

CHAPTER 5 – NADI PARIKSHAN IN CLINICAL PRACTICE

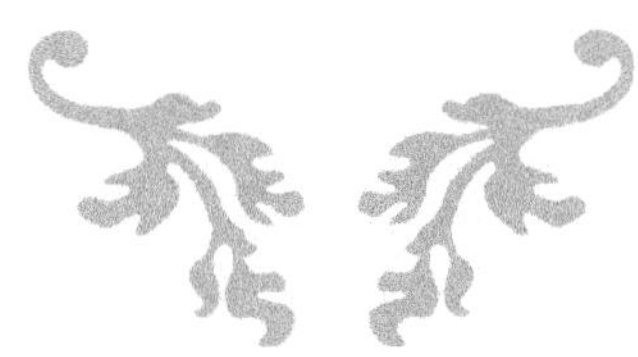

5.1 Pulse Examination in Disease Diagnosis

Pulse examination, or Nadi Parikshan, is a vital diagnostic tool in Ayurveda that provides deep insights into an individual's health by allowing practitioners to assess the balance and imbalance of the doshas—Vata, Pitta, and Kapha—within the body. By examining the pulse's characteristics, an experienced practitioner can identify potential diseases and health conditions even before they manifest physically. This proactive approach embodies the preventive and holistic nature of Ayurveda.

The Role of Pulse Examination

Pulse examination serves as a non-invasive, insightful, and efficient method for diagnosing a wide array of physiological conditions. It provides a snapshot of the body's current state, offering clues about how diseases might be developing. This enables the practitioner to address underlying imbalances before they evolve into more serious conditions.

Process of Pulse Examination for Disease Diagnosis

1. Initial Assessment:

 - The practitioner conducts the pulse reading by placing their index, middle, and ring fingers on the radial artery of the patient's wrist.

 - Each finger is responsible for gauging a specific dosha: the index for Vata, the middle for Pitta, and the ring for Kapha.

2. Evaluating Pulse Qualities:

- Rate: Variations in pulse rate can indicate underlying issues such as stress, hormonal imbalances, or cardiovascular problems.
- Rhythm: An irregular rhythm may point to potential neurological or metabolic disorders.
- Force: The strength of the pulse can reveal conditions related to cardiac health or blood pressure.
- Temperature: The warmth or coolness of the pulse site may suggest inflammatory conditions or circulation issues.

3. Identifying Dosha Imbalances:
- Vata Imbalance: May present as a light, irregular, and rapid pulse, suggesting conditions related to anxiety, insomnia, or joint issues.
- Pitta Imbalance: A sharp, intense, and warm pulse might indicate inflammatory conditions, skin disorders, or digestive issues.
- Kapha Imbalance: A heavy, slow, and steady pulse may be associated with congestion, obesity, or respiratory conditions.

4. Determining Dhatu (Tissue) Involvement:
- Practitioners use pulse characteristics to gauge the health of the body's dhatus (tissues), ensuring they receive proper nourishment and are free from disease.

5. Integrating Pulse with Other Diagnostic Measures:
- Pulse findings are combined with physical examination, patient history, and other diagnostic methods (e.g., tongue examination, eye observation) to form a comprehensive diagnosis.

Application in Specific Disease Diagnosis

- Cardiovascular Disorders:
  - Pulse examination can help detect arrhythmias, hypertension, and potential circulatory problems through irregular rhythms and force variations.

- Metabolic Conditions:
  - A rapid or irregular pulse may indicate metabolic syndromes such as diabetes or thyroid disorders, prompting further investigation.

- Digestive Disorders:
  - Variations in pulse strength and heat can point to digestive issues such as indigestion, hyperacidity, or liver disorders.

- Respiratory and Allergic Conditions:
  - A heavy, slow pulse in conjunction with cool, moist qualities may suggest respiratory congestion or allergic reactions.

- Psychological and Neurological Conditions:
  - Rapid, erratic pulses can hint at psychological stress, anxiety, or nervous system imbalances.

Limitations and Considerations

While pulse examination is a powerful tool, it requires significant expertise and experience to interpret accurately. Each individual's pulse carries unique nuances, and its characteristics can be influenced by external factors such as diet, activity, and environmental conditions. Practitioners must consider these variables and corroborate pulse findings with additional assessment methods.

Pulse examination is a cornerstone of Ayurvedic diagnostic practice, offering an in-depth understanding of the body's internal state and potential disease progression. By identifying imbalances early, practitioners can initiate personalized treatment plans that prevent disease escalation, promote balance, and support holistic health. This proactive and integrative approach aligns with Ayurveda's foundational principles, emphasizing prevention, individualized care, and the interconnectedness of the body, mind, and spirit.

5.2 Pulse Reading on Common Ailments

Pulse reading, or Nadi Parikshan, is an essential component of Ayurvedic diagnostics, offering critical insights into the health of an individual and providing early indicators of various common ailments. Through skilled assessment of the pulse's rate, rhythm, force, and other qualities, practitioners can detect imbalances in the doshas—Vata, Pitta, and Kapha—and related physiological disruptions that manifest as common health issues. Below is an in-depth exploration of how pulse reading contributes to diagnosing several prevalent conditions.

Common Ailments and Their Pulse Manifestations

1. Anxiety and Stress

- Pulse Characteristics:

- Vata Imbalance: The pulse is often rapid, irregular, and light. This reflects the erratic and anxious qualities attributed to an aggravated Vata.
- Cool and Erratic Beat: The pulse may feel cool and show an irregular rhythm with occasional missed beats, indicating nervous tension.

- Diagnosis Insight:
- This pulse pattern commonly mirrors states of excessive mental activity, worry, and stress, suggesting that therapeutic strategies should focus on stabilizing Vata through grounding and soothing practices.

2. Hypertension (High Blood Pressure)

- Pulse Characteristics:
- Pitta Predominance: The pulse may be forceful, bounding, and moderately fast. This indicates the intense and heated qualities of Pitta.
- Warmth and Sharp Beat: A noticeable warmth and sharpness in the pulse suggest an inflamed cardiovascular state.

- Diagnosis Insight:
- A forceful and heated pulse aligns with hypertension, often necessitating interventions aimed at cooling Pitta, reducing stress, and promoting relaxation.

3. Digestive Disorders

- Pulse Characteristics:

- Pitta or Vata Imbalance: In conditions like hyperacidity, ulcer, or indigestion, the pulse may present rapid, sharp qualities or an erratic Vata rhythm combined with Pitta heat.

  - Irregular and Fast: Digestive imbalances often reflect in a fast, irregular pulse, indicating metabolic disturbances or digestive fire (Agni) imbalances.

- Diagnosis Insight:

  - Therapeutic focus may include harmonizing Agni, correcting diet, and using herbs that calm Pitta or balance Vata to restore digestive health.

4. Respiratory Issues (Asthma, Allergies)

- Pulse Characteristics:

  - Kapha and Vata Disruption: The pulse may show a slow, heavy quality indicative of Kapha congestion, alongside erratic Vata influences.

  - Moist and Heavy Beat: A heavy, moist pulse suggests respiratory mucus accumulation or allergic reactions.

- Diagnosis Insight:

  - Pulse findings guide the need for therapies that clear Kapha (mucus), stabilize breathing through Vata pacification, and support respiratory function.

5. Diabetes Mellitus

- Pulse Characteristics:

  - Kapha and Pitta Imbalance: The pulse can be seen as heavy, steady, or sometimes sharp and warm due to Pitta contribution.

- Sluggish and Full: A sluggish, steady pulse with warmth may signify metabolic dysfunction related to sugar regulation.

- Diagnosis Insight:
  - Ayurvedic management will focus on dietary adjustment, enhancing digestive metabolism to process sugars effectively, and promoting healthy lifestyle habits.

6. Depression and Lethargy

- Pulse Characteristics:
  - Kapha Dominance: The pulse is typically slow, deep, and heavy, reflecting the stasis and heaviness of increased Kapha.
  - Dull and Cool: A dull pulse with coolness aligns with emotional stagnation and lethargy.

- Diagnosis Insight:
  - Treatment strategies may employ stimulating activities, dynamic herbs, and diet changes to uplift the psyche and restore vitality, reducing Kapha's heaviness.

7. Insomnia

- Pulse Characteristics:
  - Vata Imbalance: The pulse might be fast, light, and irregular, indicating heightened nervous activity and restlessness associated with Vata.
  - Weak and Erratic Beat: The pulse could feel weak and erratic, reflecting disturbed mental tranquility and sleep patterns.

- Diagnosis Insight:

- This pattern suggests a need for calming and grounding Vata through warm, nourishing routines, relaxation techniques, and herbs that promote restful sleep.

8. Irritable Bowel Syndrome (IBS)

- Pulse Characteristics:
  - Vata and Pitta Fluctuation: The pulse may show rapid changes, with sharp Pitta qualities or irregular Vata characteristics.
  - Warm and Unsteady: A warm, unsteady pulse can indicate digestive sensitivity and intestinal irritation.

- Diagnosis Insight:
  - Focus on diet adjustments, stress reduction, and supporting digestive balance, addressing both Vata's irregularity and Pitta's inflammation.

9. Rheumatoid Arthritis

- Pulse Characteristics:
  - Vata and Pitta Imbalance: The pulse can be rapid and irregular (Vata), with underlying heat and inflammation (Pitta).
  - Sharp and Light: A sharp, light pulse might suggest joint inflammation and pain, key symptoms of rheumatoid conditions.

- Diagnosis Insight:
  - Treatment may involve detoxification, joint lubrication, inflammation reduction, and calming therapies for both Vata and Pitta.

10. Sinusitis and Chronic Colds

- Pulse Characteristics:
  - Kapha Predominance: The pulse often feels sluggish and heavy, indicating Kapha congestion in the sinuses.
  - Cool and Full: Full, cool qualities in the pulse suggest mucus accumulation and fluid retention in sinuses.

- Diagnosis Insight:
  - Encouraging Kapha reduction through diet, lifestyle changes, and decongesting herbs and therapies to clear sinus blocks.

11. Acne and Skin Disorders

- Pulse Characteristics:
  - Pitta Imbalance: The pulse may be sharp and warm, reflecting excess heat and toxins affecting the skin.
  - Moderate Force: A moderately forceful pulse could point to Pitta-induced inflammatory skin conditions.

- Diagnosis Insight:
  - Management involves cooling and detoxifying Pitta, including dietary adjustments, topical treatments, and anti-inflammatory herbs.

12. Hypothyroidism

- Pulse Characteristics:
  - Kapha and Vata Imbalance: The pulse might be slow and deep, indicative of decreased metabolic function typical of Kapha imbalance.

- Dull and Cold: A cold, sluggish feeling in the pulse might suggest hypothyroid conditions affecting metabolism.

- Diagnosis Insight:
  - Treatment focuses on stimulating metabolism, supporting thyroid function, and addressing both Vata and Kapha imbalances through appropriate treatments.

13. Gastritis and Ulcers

- Pulse Characteristics:
  - Pitta Excess: A rapid, strong, and hot pulse often mirrors increased gastric acid and inflammation.
  - Sharp Beat: A sharp, aggressive pulse highlights irritation in the digestive tract due to inflammation or ulcers.

- Diagnosis Insight:
  - Cooling Pitta through food choices, stress management, and specific herbal supplements helps manage these conditions.

14. Menstrual Disorders (e.g., Dysmenorrhea, Amenorrhea)

- Pulse Characteristics:
  - Vata and Pitta Fluctuation: The pulse may be irregular and rapid, reflecting the hormonal and systemic imbalances.
  - Unsteady and Warm: Possible unsteady, warm qualities in the pulse suggest disruption in reproductive or menstrual cycles.

- Diagnosis Insight:
  - Addressing hormonal balance through lifestyle changes, herbal remedies, and dietary support aimed at balancing Vata and Pitta.

15. Obesity

- Pulse Characteristics:
  - Kapha Predominance: The pulse is typically slow, heavy, and full, reflecting Kapha's qualities of heaviness and accumulation.
  - Steady and Cool: A steady, cool pulse suggests sluggish metabolism and lethargy characteristic of excess Kapha.

- Diagnosis Insight:
  - Encourage metabolism stimulation, promote activity, and employ dietary strategies to balance Kapha and reduce bodyweight naturally.

16. Chronic Fatigue Syndrome

- Pulse Characteristics:
  - Vata and Kapha Imbalance: The pulse may be weak, light, and slightly erratic, indicating diminished vitality and exhaustion.
  - Weak and Unstable: Displaying instability and weakness, the pulse conveys systemic fatigue and depletion of energy reserves.

- Diagnosis Insight:
  - Focus on rejuvenation therapies, stress management, and dietary and lifestyle modifications to balance Vata and Kapha, restoring energy levels.

17. Osteoarthritis

- Pulse Characteristics:

- Vata Predominance: The pulse often presents with a rough, light, and irregular quality, indicating deteriorating joint health.
 - Weak and Dry: A weak, dry pulse may point to joint degeneration and lack of lubrication typical of Vata imbalances.

- Diagnosis Insight:
 - Emphasize therapies that lubricate joints, improve flexibility, and soothe Vata imbalances to alleviate joint degeneration symptoms.

18. Urinary Tract Infections (UTIs)

- Pulse Characteristics:
 - Pitta and Kapha Imbalance: The pulse may be sharp, warm, and moist, indicating inflammation and infection.
 - Warm and Heavy: Displays heat and moisture, aligned with Kapha's accumulation and inflammatory processes.

- Diagnosis Insight:
 - Cooling, astringent, and diuretic herbs alongside hydration and hygiene practices aim to pacify Pitta and manage UTIs effectively.

19. Migraines and Chronic Headaches

- Pulse Characteristics:
 - Vata and Pitta Fluctuation: The pulse can be rapid, sharp, and sometimes erratic, suggesting vascular and neurological tension.
 - Sharp and Rapid Beat: Indicates active Pitta overheating, often combined with Vata's erratic nature causing pain perception.

- Diagnosis Insight:

- Provide cooling and calming strategies, leveraging appropriate herbal interventions to resolve headache triggers from Pitta and Vata influence.

20. Hyperthyroidism

- Pulse Characteristics:
  - Pitta and Vata Imbalance: The pulse may feel rapid, strong, and with pronounced warmth, indicating metabolic hyperactivity.
  - Rapid and Hot: Exhibiting heat and speed, the pulse reflects an overactive thyroid function and high energy expenditure.

- Diagnosis Insight:
  - Cooling, grounding treatments that stabilize metabolism and calm excessive energy output, realigning Pitta and Vata within balance.

21. Constipation

- Pulse Characteristics:
  - Vata Disruption: The pulse is often light, irregular, and weak, indicating digestive irregularity and dryness.
  - Weak and Erratic: Expressions of irregular Vata disruption seen in slow or incomplete evacuation patterns.

- Diagnosis Insight:
  - Emphasize lubrication, soothing regimens, and digestive stimulants to support regular bowel movements and Vata balance.

22. Skin Rashes and Allergies

- Pulse Characteristics:
  - Pitta and Kapha Imbalance: Warmth, sharpness, and possible heaviness in the pulse indicate inflammatory skin manifestations.
  - Warm and Sharp Beat: Reflects redness, swelling, and irritation correlated with heightened Pitta and Kapha influences.

- Diagnosis Insight:
  - Focus on cooling, cleansing, and anti-inflammatory protocols to clear toxins, purify the blood, and restore skin health.

Integrative Diagnosis and Treatment

While pulse reading is a profound diagnostic tool, it works best in combination with other assessments such as patient interviews, observation, and lifestyle analysis. Ayurvedic practitioners synthesize this information to formulate holistic, individualized treatment plans that target the root causes of ailments.

Understanding the pulse in the context of common ailments enables Ayurvedic practitioners to adopt a proactive approach to health, addressing imbalances early and supporting the body's innate healing processes. This comprehensive methodology not only alleviates symptoms but also seeks to restore and maintain equilibrium in body, mind, and spirit, embodying Ayurveda's holistic and preventive health philosophy.

5.3 Monitoring Patient Progress Through Pulse

In Ayurveda, continuous monitoring of a patient's progress is essential to ensure the effectiveness and appropriateness of the treatment plan. Pulse examination, or Nadi Parikshan, serves as a dynamic tool for tracking changes in the patient's health status over time. This ongoing assessment allows practitioners to make informed adjustments to interventions and therapies, ultimately supporting the patient's journey toward balance and well-being.

The Role of Pulse Examination in Monitoring Progress
Pulse examination captures the subtle shifts in doshic balance and other physiological factors, providing a real-time picture of the individual's internal state. By regularly evaluating pulse characteristics, practitioners can:

1. Assess Treatment Efficacy:
   - Determine how well the current interventions are addressing the patient's conditions and goals. A positive response is often reflected in pulse qualities that move toward equilibrium — steady rhythms, balanced temperatures, and harmonious depths.

2. Detect Emerging Imbalances:
   - Early identification of new or recurring imbalances allows for timely modifications to treatment strategies, preventing potential deterioration or complications.

3. Guide Therapeutic Adjustments:

- Each pulse characteristic guides nuanced adjustments in diet, lifestyle, herbal remedies, and therapies, ensuring they remain aligned with the individual's evolving state.

Key Parameters for Monitoring Through Pulse

1. Rate and Rhythm Adjustments:

- Rate: An improvement in disorders associated with high Vata or Pitta may show as a normalization of pulse rate, with a slower, more balanced beat indicating reduced stress, anxiety, or inflammation.

- Rhythm: A regular rhythm replacing irregular Vata pulses suggests stabilization in nervous system function and mental coherence.

2. Dosha-specific Changes:

- Pulse Shifts for Vata: Enhanced Vata balance reveals itself in a steadier, more grounded pulse, showing improved energy levels and reduced erratic symptoms.

- Pulse Shifts for Pitta: A cooling down of sharp, intense pulse characteristics signals a decrease in Pitta-related conditions like inflammation or excessive heat.

- Pulse Shifts for Kapha: The pulse may become lighter and more dynamic as Kapha conditions improve, reflecting decreased heaviness and fluid accumulation.

3. Temperature and Volume Modifications:

- Temperature: A balanced temperature in the pulse highlights effective cooling or warming therapies, depending on whether Pitta or Kapha imbalances are being addressed.

- Volume: Adjustments in pulse volume can denote changes in systemic or circulatory health, including improvements in circulation and heart function through appropriate therapy.

4. Complexity and Depth:
- Complexity: The transition from complex, combined pulse qualities to simpler, more defined patterns signals the resolution of layered imbalances in the patient's health.
- Depth: A pulse moving toward appropriate depths—neither excessively superficial nor deep—shows healthy tissue function and dosha equilibrium.

Practical Application

1. Regular Check-ups:
   - Incorporate pulse checks during each consultation to establish a comparable baseline that reflects patient progress over time.

2. Documentation:
   - Keep detailed records of pulse characteristics during each visit, noting any correlations between pulse changes and reported symptoms or improvements.

3. Patient Involvement:
   - Educate patients on how lifestyle practices and home routines influence their pulse and overall health, fostering proactive engagement in their own healing process.

4. Interdisciplinary Coordination:
   - Pulse findings may complement modern diagnostic methods, allowing for an enriched understanding of the patient's evolving conditions.

Monitoring patient progress through pulse examination is a powerful approach deeply rooted in Ayurvedic tradition. This practice offers continuous feedback on the patient's journey towards balance, enabling the effective adaptation of therapies to meet their unique needs.

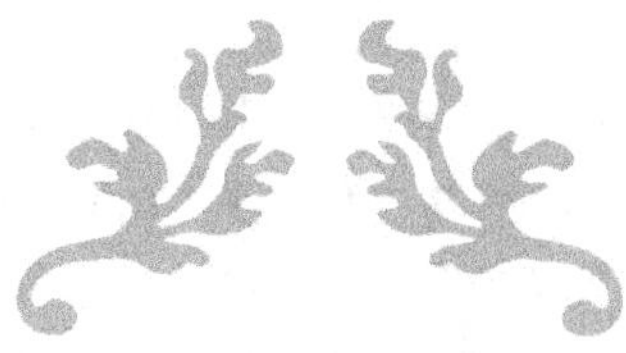

CHAPTER 6 –
COMPLIMENTARY
AYURVEDA
THERAPIES

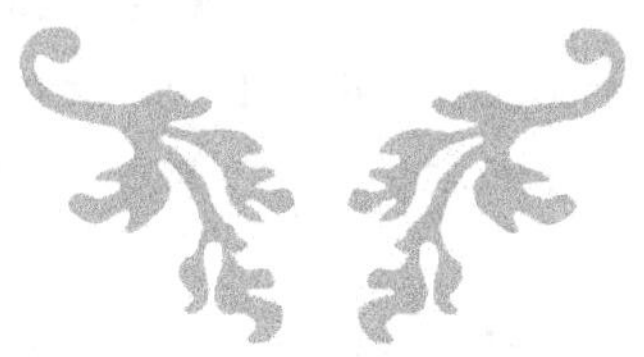

6.1 Panchakarma and Its Role in Balance Restoration

Panchakarma is a cornerstone therapeutic practice in Ayurveda, renowned for its profound ability to cleanse the body, restore balance, and enhance overall health. Derived from the Sanskrit words "Pancha," meaning five, and "Karma," meaning actions or processes, Panchakarma consists of five major procedures aimed at detoxifying and rejuvenating the body and mind. This ancient practice is pivotal in resetting the body's natural balance, thereby cultivating health, vitality, and longevity.

The Objectives and Benefits of Panchakarma

The primary objective of Panchakarma is to eliminate accumulated toxins (ama) and balance the tridoshas—Vata, Pitta, and Kapha. The benefits of such purification are extensive:

- Detoxification: Removal of deep-seated toxins and impurities that can obstruct physiological functions and lead to disease.
- Revitalization: Rejuvenates the body's tissues, improving strength, immunity, and vitality.
- Balance Restoration: Restores doshic balance within the body, addressing specific imbalances that contribute to health issues.
- Mental Clarity: Enhances mental clarity, emotional stability, and overall well-being by removing psychological toxins and promoting relaxation.
- Prevention and Disease Management: Helps in the prevention of diseases and supports management of chronic conditions by addressing root causes through systemic purification.

The Five Core Procedures of Panchakarma

Panchakarma involves five primary cleansing techniques, each targeting specific systems and functions within the body. These procedures are often customized based on the individual's constitution (Prakriti), dosha imbalances (Vikriti), and specific health concerns.

1. Vamana (Therapeutic Emesis):
  - Purpose: Induces vomiting to expel excessive Kapha, especially from the respiratory and gastrointestinal systems.
  - Benefits: Effective in treating conditions like asthma, chronic colds, allergies, and digestive disorders associated with Kapha accumulation.

2. Virechana (Therapeutic Purgation):
  - Purpose: Utilizes natural laxatives to cleanse the small intestine and liver, targeting excess Pitta dosha.
  - Benefits: Addresses skin disorders, hyperacidity, jaundice, and inflammatory conditions by cooling and purifying the body.

3. Basti (Medicated Enema):
  - Purpose: Administers herbal oils and decoctions via the rectum to eliminate Vata-related toxins.
  - Benefits: Especially beneficial for arthritis, constipation, neurological disorders, and other Vata-induced conditions by nourishing and lubricating the colon.

4. Nasya (Nasal Administration):
  - Purpose: Introduces medicated oils or powders through the nasal passages, purifying head and neck regions.
  - Benefits: Addresses sinusitis, migraines, allergies, and mental stress by clearing respiratory passages and enhancing mental clarity.

5. Raktamokshana (Bloodletting):
   - Purpose: Removes impure blood to treat diseases caused by
blood impurities, focusing on Pitta-related disorders.
   - Benefits: Effective for skin conditions, hypertension, and other
inflammatory ailments by reducing excess heat and toxins in the
blood.

Supporting Procedures and Preparatory Steps
Panchakarma requires careful preparation and follow-up to
maximize its efficacy:

- Purvakarma (Preparation): Involves practices like Snehana
(oleation) and Swedana (sudation) to lubricate and loosen toxins,
making their elimination easier.
- Paschatkarma (Post-therapy Care): Includes dietary
adjustments, rest, and specific lifestyle recommendations to
facilitate recovery and maintain balance.
- Rejuvenation (Rasayana): Post-cleansing therapies and herbal
preparations that support tissue regeneration and immune
strengthening.

The Role of Panchakarma in Modern Health
In modern health contexts, Panchakarma draws interest as an
effective complementary therapy, integrating traditional wisdom
with contemporary health practices. Its efficacy in managing
chronic diseases, promoting detoxification, and enhancing
mental well-being makes it an asset in integrative medicine.

Panchakarma offers a profound pathway to restoring balance and
health, representing the holistic nature of Ayurvedic healing. By
systematically removing physical and mental toxins, it revitalizes

the body, fosters emotional equilibrium, and prepares individuals for sustained health and spiritual growth. Its tailored application underscores Ayurveda's commitment to individualized care, enabling personal transformation and the cultivation of well-being at its deepest level.

6.2 Herbal Remedies and Their Pulse Implications

In Ayurveda, herbal remedies play an instrumental role in restoring balance and health. These remedies are meticulously chosen based on their properties and their ability to influence the doshas—Vata, Pitta, and Kapha. By carefully assessing the pulse through Nadi Parikshan, practitioners can identify doshic imbalances and prescribe appropriate herbal treatments. Understanding the implications of these remedies on the pulse is crucial in ensuring the effectiveness of Ayurvedic intervention.

The Pulse and Herbal Remedies

The pulse acts as a diagnostic gateway, providing insights into the current state of doshas and any imbalances present. Once a doshic imbalance is identified through pulse diagnosis, specific herbs are chosen to correct these imbalances. Monitoring pulse changes after administering herbal remedies allows practitioners to gauge the effectiveness of the treatment and make necessary adjustments.

<u>6.2 Herbal Remedies and Their Impact on the Pulse</u>

Herbs for Vata Imbalance

1. Ashwagandha (Withania somnifera):
   - Properties: Adaptogenic, grounding, nervine tonic.
   - Pulse Implications: Ashwagandha helps stabilize and strengthen a weak, erratic Vata pulse by grounding and nourishing the nervous system, often resulting in a steadier and more rhythmically sound pulse.

2. Bala (Sida cordifolia):
   - Properties: Strengthening, rejuvenating, anti-inflammatory.
   - Pulse Implications: Known to nourish and stabilize, Bala can help transform a light, irregular pulse into one that is more grounded and consistent, reflecting improved Vata stability.

3. Punarnava (Boerhavia diffusa):
   - Properties: Diuretic, rejuvenative, anti-inflammatory.
   - Pulse Implications: Punarnava aids in reducing a heavy and slow Kapha pulse by supporting kidney function and fluid balance, enhancing a lighter, more dynamic pulse.

4. Pippali (Piper longum):
   - Properties: Digestive stimulant, respiratory enhancer, rejuvenating.
   - Pulse Implications: Pippali invigorates a sluggish and cool Kapha pulse by enhancing metabolism and clearing respiratory blockages, leading to an increased vitality reflected in the pulse.

5. Guggulu (Commiphora mukul):
   - Properties: Anti-inflammatory, detoxifying, rejuvenative.
   - Pulse Implications: Guggulu helps transform a weak, irregular Vata pulse by enhancing circulation and reducing inflammation, leading to a more stable and robust pulse reflective of improved joint and tissue health.

6. Valerian (Valeriana officinalis):
   - Properties: Sedative, calming, sleep aid.
   - Pulse Implications: Valerian moderates an erratic and fast Vata pulse due to its calming effects, resulting in a steadier and more regular rhythm, indicating reduced anxiety and improved relaxation.

7. Hibiscus (Hibiscus rosa-sinensis):
   - Properties: Moisturizing, cooling, calming.
   - Pulse Implications: Hibiscus can help stabilize a rapid, irregular Vata pulse by providing moisture and calming the nervous system, resulting in a more consistent and rhythmic beat.

8. Hawthorn Berry (Crataegus laevigata):
   - Properties: Cardiovascular tonic, anxiolytic, antioxidant.
   - Pulse Implications: Known to strengthen and regularize heart function, Hawthorn Berry can transform a weak, erratic Vata pulse into a more stable and rhythmic pattern, reflecting improved cardiovascular health.

Herbs for Pitta Imbalance

1. Brahmi (Bacopa monnieri):
   - Properties: Cooling, calming, cognitive enhancer.
   - Pulse Implications: Brahmi's cooling effect can transform a hot, intense Pitta pulse into a cooler, more balanced rhythm, indicating reduced Pitta agitation and inflammation.

2. Guduchi (Tinospora cordifolia):
   - Properties: Detoxifying, anti-inflammatory, immune-boosting.

   - Pulse Implications: Guduchi can moderate the intensity and heat of a Pitta pulse, leading to a reduction in excess heat and contributing to a more even and calm pulse.

3. Neem (Azadirachta indica):
   - Properties: Cooling, detoxifying, antifungal.
   - Pulse Implications: Neem's cooling nature helps temper an intense and fast Pitta pulse, transforming it into a cooler and more balanced rhythm, indicative of detoxification and reduced inflammation.

4. Amla (Emblica officinalis):
   - Properties: Antioxidant, cooling, rejuvenative.
   - Pulse Implications: Amla's cooling and revitalizing properties can lower the heat in a Pitta pulse, leading to a steadier, more moderate pulse, demonstrating reduced oxidative stress and heat.

5. Sandalwood (Santalum album):
   - Properties: Cooling, calming, anti-inflammatory.
   - Pulse Implications: Sandalwood's cooling nature can temper a sharp, warm Pitta pulse, leading to a more moderate and balanced beat, reflecting reduced heat and stress within the body.

6. Anantamul (Hemidesmus indicus):
   - Properties: Blood purifier, cooling, anti-inflammatory.
   - Pulse Implications: Anantamul helps lower the intensity of a Pitta pulse through its detoxifying effects, resulting in a cooler, less forceful pulse indicative of purified blood and reduced inflammation.

7. Manjistha (Rubia cordifolia):
   - Properties: Blood purifier, anti-inflammatory, cooling.
   - Pulse Implications: Manjistha can cool and purify the blood, helping to moderate a hot, rapid Pitta pulse by leading to a cooler, more balanced beat, indicative of reduced inflammation and detoxification.

8. Coriander (Coriandrum sativum):
   - Properties: Digestive stimulant, cooling, anti-inflammatory.
   - Pulse Implications: Coriander helps cool a sharp Pitta pulse, yielding a more moderate pulse rhythm that suggests effective digestion and reduced digestive fire.

Herbs for Kapha Imbalance

1. Trikatu (Combination of Black Pepper, Long Pepper, and Ginger):
   - Properties: Digestive stimulant, metabolism enhancer, Kapha-reducing.
   - Pulse Implications: By stimulating metabolism, Trikatu can lighten a sluggish, heavy Kapha pulse, resulting in a more dynamic and lively rhythm.

2. Guggulu (Commiphora mukul):
   - Properties: Anti-inflammatory, lipid-lowering, detoxifying.
   - Pulse Implications: Guggulu helps to invigorate the system, turning a slow, full Kapha pulse into one exhibiting increased vitality and circulation.

3. Shatavari (Asparagus racemosus):
   - Properties: Nourishing, adaptogenic, hormonal balancer.

- Pulse Implications: Shatavari helps to stabilize a weak and irregular Vata pulse by providing moisture and strength, leading to a more grounded and consistent pulse, often reflecting improved hormonal and nervous system support.

4. Licorice (Glycyrrhiza glabra):
   - Properties: Demulcent, harmonizing, anti-inflammatory.
   - Pulse Implications: Licorice's soothing qualities enhance a dry and erratic Vata pulse, resulting in a fuller, more steady beat that suggests restored hydration and systemic calmness.

5. Mustard seed (Brassica juncea):
   - Properties: Stimulant, expectorant, carminative.
   - Pulse Implications: Mustard seed can invigorate a slow, heavy Kapha pulse by enhancing metabolism and clearing respiratory pathways, resulting in a lighter, more active pulse.

6. Bay leaf (Laurus nobilis):
   - Properties: Digestive aid, anti-inflammatory, respiratory booster.
   - Pulse Implications: Bay leaf assists in lightening a Kapha pulse by stimulating digestive fire and reducing congestion, reflecting improved digestion and metabolic activity.

7. Eucalyptus (Eucalyptus globulus):
   - Properties: Respiratory stimulant, expectorant, antimicrobial.
   - Pulse Implications: Eucalyptus can invigorate a slow Kapha pulse by promoting respiratory function and metabolism, resulting in a lighter and more dynamic pulse.

8. Fenugreek (Trigonella foenum-graecum):

- Properties: Digestive aid, anti-inflammatory, metabolic booster.
- Pulse Implications: By stimulating digestion and metabolism, Fenugreek can help lighten and activate a heavy, slow Kapha pulse, reflecting improved tissue transformation and fluid balance.

Monitoring Pulse Changes with Herbal Treatments

- Before Treatment: Initial pulse diagnosis helps identify which doshas are predominant or imbalanced, guiding the choice of appropriate herbs.
- During Treatment: Regular monitoring of the pulse allows practitioners to observe changes and ensure that the treatment is moving the pulse qualities toward balance.
- After Treatment: A well-adjusted pulse that aligns with the individual's Prakriti (natural constitution) indicates successful treatment. Any necessary adjustments are made based on lingering imbalances detected in the pulse.

Integrative Approach

In addition to the pulse implications of specific herbs, the broader context in which these herbs are used includes lifestyle and dietary recommendations that support the healing process. Practitioners take a holistic view, integrating pulse readings, herb properties, lifestyle factors, and patient feedback to tailor treatment plans effectively.

The integration of herbal remedies with pulse diagnosis in Ayurveda is a testament to the system's comprehensive and personalized approach to healing. By bridging the insights gained through Nadi Parikshan with the targeted effects of herbal treatments, Ayurvedic practitioners can facilitate profound shifts toward balance and wellness. This synergy not only addresses physical symptoms but also harmonizes the underlying doshic imbalances, promoting enhanced vitality and overall health.

6.3 Lifestyle Modifications Based on Pulse Readings

In Ayurveda, lifestyle plays a crucial role in maintaining health and balance among the doshas—Vata, Pitta, and Kapha. Pulse readings, or Nadi Parikshan, provide insights into an individual's constitution and current doshic imbalances, making it possible for practitioners to recommend specific lifestyle modifications that support well-being. Tailoring daily routines to align with these findings can significantly enhance health outcomes and promote a harmonious balance within the body and mind.

Lifestyle Modifications for Vata Imbalance

When a pulse reading indicates Vata imbalance, characterized by lightness, irregular rhythms, and coolness, the following lifestyle adjustments can help stabilize Vata:

1. Daily Routine:

   - Establish regular daily routines with consistent meal times and sleep schedules to provide grounding and stability to the erratic nature of Vata.

2. Dietary Adjustments:

   - Consume warm, cooked foods rich in good fats and oils, such as soups, stews, and warm grains like oatmeal. Incorporate spices like ginger and cinnamon to aid digestion and warmth.

3. Physical Activity:

- Engage in grounding and calming exercises such as yoga, tai chi, or gentle walking. Avoid overly stimulating or high-intensity workouts that can increase Vata's imbalance.

4. Mindfulness Practices:
   - Integrate mindfulness and relaxation practices such as meditation, deep breathing, and grounding techniques to reduce anxiety and mental chatter.

Lifestyle Modifications for Pitta Imbalance

For individuals with a Pitta imbalance highlighted by a hot, intense pulse, cooling and calming measures can mitigate excess Pitta:

1. Daily Routine:
   - Incorporate periods of rest and avoid over-scheduling to reduce stress and prevent burnout. Aim for balance between activity and relaxation.

2. Dietary Adjustments:
   - Favor cooling, refreshing foods like cucumbers, melons, and leafy greens. Reduce spicy, acidic, and fried foods that increase heat. Use cooling herbs like cilantro and mint.

3. Physical Activity:
   - Opt for outdoor activities during cooler parts of the day, such as swimming or gentle cycling, to release heat. Avoid competitive or aggressive sports that can exacerbate Pitta.

4. Mindfulness Practices:

- Practice cooling breathwork like Sitali Pranayama and engage in calming meditations to soothe intensity and foster emotional balance.

Lifestyle Modifications for Kapha Imbalance

Kapha imbalance, reflected in a heavy, slow pulse, benefits from invigorating and stimulating adjustments to reduce heaviness and promote movement:

1. Daily Routine:

  - Break up the routine with varied activities and ensure a stimulating environment to counteract lethargy. Wake up early to harness morning energy.

2. Dietary Adjustments:

  - Incorporate light, dry foods and warming spices that stimulate digestion, such as chili, black pepper, and turmeric. Limit dairy, sweets, and oily foods.

3. Physical Activity:

  - Engage in regular exercise that energizes and heats the body, like jogging, aerobics, or dance. Aim for consistent physical activity to maintain lightness.

4. Mindfulness Practices:

  - Practice energizing breathing techniques such as Kapalabhati and participate in lively, dynamic activities that uplift the spirit and promote vitality.

Comprehensive and Personalized Approach

These lifestyle modifications are designed to align with an individual's unique doshic constitution and pulse findings. The personalized approach ensures that recommendations not only address symptoms but also target root causes of imbalances, promoting a comprehensive path to wellness.

By integrating lifestyle adjustments based on pulse readings, Ayurvedic practitioners empower individuals to take an active role in their own health management. These modifications, informed by the nuances of pulse diagnosis, foster a harmonious living environment that supports balance and holistic well-being. The approach underscores Ayurveda's commitment to individualized care, promoting long-term health and resilience through practical and meaningful daily practices.

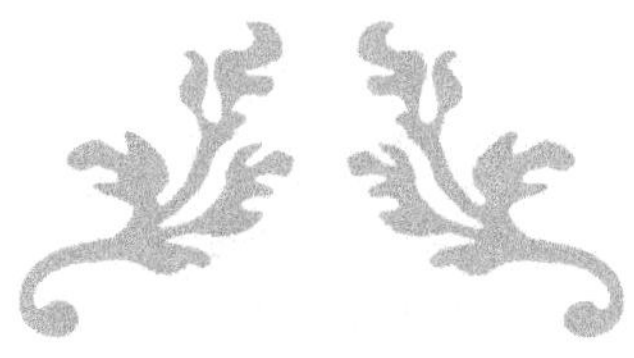

CHAPTER 7 – INTEGRATION WITH MORDERN MEDICINE

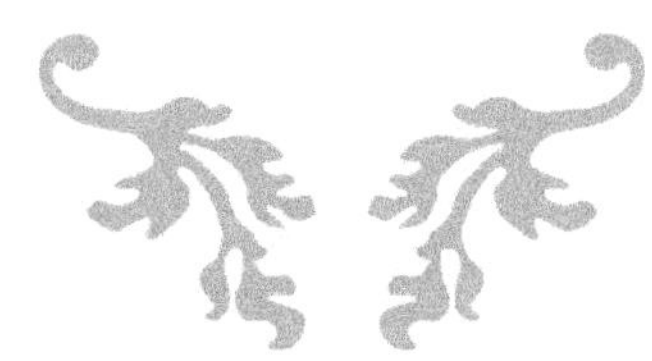

7.1 Modern Scientific Perspective on Pulse Examination

Pulse examination has been an essential diagnostic tool in traditional medical systems such as Ayurveda and Traditional Chinese Medicine for centuries. With the advent of modern scientific inquiry, there has been increasing interest in exploring and validating the physiological basis and diagnostic potential of pulse reading. This exploration offers promising intersections between ancient wisdom and contemporary biomedical understanding.

Physiological Basis of Pulse

The pulse, in a biomedical context, is the tactile arterial palpation of the heartbeat by trained fingertips. It is most examined at the radial artery near the wrist but can also be assessed at various other points, such as the carotid artery in the neck or brachial artery in the arm. The pulse provides crucial information about:

1. Heart Rate: The number of pulse beats per minute, offering insights into the cardiovascular and systemic health.

2. Rhythm: Regularity of the pulse which can indicate normal cardiac function or arrhythmias.

3. Strength and Volume: Can suggest cardiac output and blood flow consistency.

4. Tension and Elasticity: Reflects vascular tone and health of the arterial walls.

Modern Technological Innovations

- Digital Pulse Analysis: Advanced devices have been developed to measure pulse characteristics with high precision, providing detailed information on heart rate variability, arterial stiffness, and vascular health. These devices use sensors and algorithms to analyse the pulse waveforms for diagnostic purposes.

- Wearable Technology: Smartwatches and fitness trackers monitor pulse in real-time, helping to track heart rate trends and identify anomalies that could require further medical evaluation.

- Photoplethysmography (PPG): A non-invasive method that uses a light source and a photodetector to reflect changes in blood volume, allowing the analysis of pulse waveform characteristics and offering insights into cardiovascular function.

"Nadi Tarangini"

"Nadi Tarangini" is an innovative technology developed to bring the ancient practice of Nadi Parikshan, or pulse diagnosis, into the modern era. It aims to integrate traditional Ayurvedic diagnostic methods with contemporary scientific advances, providing a more standardized and objective approach to pulse analysis.

Developed by eminent innovators in India, Nadi Tarangini uses modern sensors and software algorithms to capture, analyse, and interpret pulse signals. This system bridges the gap between subjective expert assessment in traditional Nadi Parikshan and the requirements for precision and consistency in modern medical diagnostics.

Key Features

1. Sensor Technology:

- Nadi Tarangini employs specialized sensors to accurately detect pulse waveforms at the radial artery. These sensors capture the pulse with high precision, recording various aspects such as rate, rhythm, force, and patterns.

2. Data Interpretation:

   - The device processes and analyses the captured pulse data using sophisticated algorithms. This analysis considers various parameters to identify doshic imbalances and suggests potential health conditions based on the derived pulse characteristics.

3. User-Friendly Interface:

   - Equipped with a user-friendly software interface, Nadi Tarangini enables practitioners to easily review and understand the results. It provides visual interpretations of the pulse readings, which can be used to make informed decisions regarding patient diagnosis and management.

4. Integration with Health Records:

   - The system may integrate with digital health records, allowing for comprehensive patient monitoring and longitudinal health assessments. This can enhance personalized care plans and track patient progress over time.

Benefits

- Standardization: By providing a consistent and objective method for pulse diagnosis, Nadi Tarangini reduces the variability inherent in traditional pulse reading, thus enhancing reliability and credibility.

- Accessibility: The technology makes pulse analysis accessible to a broader range of practitioners, including those less experienced in traditional methods, by offering a guided, analytical approach.

- Complementary Tool: While not a replacement for expert Ayurvedic consultation, Nadi Tarangini serves as a complementary diagnostic tool that integrates traditional wisdom with modern precision, catering to both Ayurvedic and integrative medicine practitioners.

Challenges and Considerations
- Validation and Research: As with any new medical technology, ongoing research and clinical validation are necessary to confirm the accuracy, reliability, and comprehensive applicability of the Nadi Tarangini system across diverse patient populations.

- Training and Adoption: Effective implementation requires training practitioners to understand and interpret the results accurately, ensuring that the technology supports rather than supplants traditional diagnostic skills.

Nadi Tarangini represents a significant advancement in the field of Ayurvedic diagnostics, offering an innovative way to unify traditional practices with contemporary technological approaches. It reflects a broader movement in integrative healthcare, where the synthesis of ancient knowledge and modern technology promises to enhance diagnostic capabilities and improve patient outcomes. By facilitating this harmony, Nadi Tarangini holds the potential to enrich the practice of Ayurveda and highlight its relevance in the modern medical landscape.

Scientific Investigations and Correlations

Research has been increasingly focused on the potential of pulse analysis as a diagnostic tool in modern medicine. Some areas of exploration include:

- Heart Rate Variability (HRV): Studied as an indicator of autonomic nervous system activity and its effects on health, showing correlations between psychological stress, wellness, and disease states.

- Arterial Stiffness Measurement: Used to assess cardiovascular health risks, with pulse wave velocity being a critical parameter for determining arterial stiffness and related health conditions.

Integration with Traditional Pulse Diagnosis

- Holistic Health Metrics: Some studies aim to correlate traditional characteristics (such as those described in Ayurvedic and Chinese medicine) with quantitative metrics in pulse analysis, seeking scientific explanations for traditional observations.

- Complementary Diagnostic Use: Pulse examination complements other diagnostic tools in clinical settings, where integrative health practitioners combine traditional insights with modern findings for a more holistic approach to patient care.

Challenges and Opportunities

- Standardization and Training: Despite technological advances, standardizing pulse diagnosis remains challenging, partially due to the subjective nature of traditional pulse reading. Clear guidelines and training are needed to improve reliability in clinical practice.

- Research and Validation: Ongoing research is required to validate the efficacy of traditional pulse diagnosis methods in modern clinical scenarios and to explore the full potential of technological advancements in pulse analysis.

The modern scientific perspective on pulse examination highlights the potential for cross-disciplinary benefits from integrating traditional pulse diagnosis with contemporary medical technology and research. By bridging the gap between ancient practices and modern science, there is a rich opportunity for enhancing diagnostic accuracy, understanding systemic health, and promoting integrative healthcare approaches. This dialogue between old and new holds the promise of developing a more comprehensive and effective diagnostic landscape that respects the wisdom of traditional medicine while leveraging the precision of modern technology.

7.2 Comparative Analysis with Modern Diagnostic Techniques

Ayurvedic Nadi Parikshan, or pulse diagnosis, has been a cornerstone of traditional medicine, offering insights into the balance of doshas—Vata, Pitta, and Kapha—and the overall health of the individual. In contrast, modern diagnostic techniques utilize advanced technology and scientific principles to analyze physiological and pathological conditions. This comparison seeks to explore both the complementary and distinctive aspects of these approaches, highlighting opportunities for integration.

Traditional Nadi Parikshan

Core Principles:

- Holistic Assessment: Focuses on the dynamic interplay of doshas and how they manifest in the body and mind, emphasizing personalized health.
- Qualitative Analysis: Relies on subjective assessment of pulse qualities like rhythm, force, temperature, and depth, which require extensive practitioner experience.
- Prevention and Early Detection: Aims to detect imbalances before symptoms manifest physically, offering preventive care insights.

Modern Diagnostic Techniques

Core Principles:

- Objective Measurement: Utilizes measurable data to assess health, emphasizing accuracy and consistency.
- Quantitative Analysis: Employs devices like blood tests, imaging (e.g., MRI, CT scans), and wearable health monitors to evaluate specific health parameters.
- Disease Identification and Management: Focuses on identifying existing conditions and managing symptoms and diseases with targeted interventions.

Comparative Analysis

1. Methodology and Approach

- Traditional Nadi Parikshan:

  - Involves the practitioner's skill in interpreting the subtle qualities of the pulse, often relying on intuition and experience.
  - Diagnostic insight is drawn from a holistic understanding of the individual's constitution and lifestyle.

- Modern Diagnostics:

- Relies heavily on reproducible and standardized measurements, ensuring consistency across different practitioners and settings.
  - Utilizes technology to obtain precise data for diagnosis, often focusing on specific anatomical or biochemical parameters.

2. Scope of Diagnosis

- Traditional Nadi Parikshan:
  - Offers a comprehensive view of the individual's current state of health, including emotional and mental well-being, by assessing doshic balance.

- Modern Diagnostics:
  - Provides detailed insights into specific organ function and pathology, using targeted tests to confirm or rule out particular medical conditions.

3. Applications and Limitations

- Traditional Nadi Parikshan:
  - Strength lies in its ability to detect subtle imbalances early, guiding preventive lifestyle and dietary changes.
  - Limitations include potential subjectivity and variability in diagnostic conclusions based on the practitioner's expertise.

- Modern Diagnostics:
  - Excels in identifying and quantifying existing health conditions, facilitating evidence-based treatment plans.
  - Limitations involve potential focus on symptomatic treatment rather than addressing underlying holistic conditions.

Opportunities for Integration

- Complementary Use: Combining Nadi Parikshan with modern diagnostics can enrich patient assessment, using traditional methods for holistic insights and modern techniques for precise, detailed analysis.

- Enhanced Preventive Care: Nadi Parikshan can guide preventive strategies, while modern diagnostics provide ongoing monitoring and validation of health interventions.

- Personalized Medicine: Both systems support the development of personalized care plans, integrating individual constitution and lifestyle considerations with targeted treatments.

By examining the complementary strengths of traditional Nadi Parikshan and modern diagnostic techniques, healthcare practitioners can craft a more comprehensive and integrative approach to patient care. This dual methodology respects the subjective and objective nature of health, fostering an environment where ancient wisdom meets modern science to enhance well-being and healing. The synergy between these systems holds promise for the advancement of personalized and preventive medicine, drawing on the best of both worlds to improve health outcomes.

7.3 Opportunities for Integrative Healthcare Practices

Integrative healthcare practices combine the ancient wisdom of traditional systems like Ayurveda with the advances of modern medical science. This holistic approach seeks to treat patients not only based on symptomatic relief but also by addressing the root causes of imbalance, considering the physical, emotional, and spiritual aspects of health. An integrative model offers many opportunities to enhance patient care by drawing from a diverse range of diagnostic and therapeutic strategies.

Key Opportunities for Integration

1. Holistic Patient Assessment
- Syncretizing Diagnostic Tools:
  - Traditional and Modern Fusion: Applying Nadi Parikshan in tandem with modern diagnostic methods such as blood tests and imaging can provide a comprehensive understanding of the patient's health. This fusion allows the recognition of subtle doshic imbalances alongside precise, data-driven physiological assessments.
  - Broadening Perspectives: By incorporating multiple diagnostic perspectives, practitioners can observe both macro and micro health dynamics, improving the depth and accuracy of diagnoses.

2. Enhanced Preventive Care
- Early Detection and Lifestyle Guidance:
  - Proactive Health Management: Through the predictive capacity of Ayurvedic methods like pulse diagnosis, integrative healthcare can encourage lifestyle and dietary changes before severe symptoms develop, reducing the risk of chronic diseases.
  - Long-term Wellness Strategies: Combining modern preventive screenings with Ayurvedic rituals, such as seasonal cleansing and rejuvenation therapy, fosters sustained health and quality of life.

3. Personalized Treatment Plans
- Customization Based on Individual Needs:
  - Tailored Therapies: Integrative practices can develop personalized care plans that align with an individual's unique

constitution (Prakriti), lifestyle, and preferences, utilizing
Ayurvedic herbs and practices alongside pharmaceutical or
surgical interventions when appropriate.

 - Interdisciplinary Collaboration: Collaborations between
Ayurvedic practitioners, general physicians, nutritionists, and
mental health professionals ensure a multilateral approach,
offering the best-suited combination of therapies for each
patient.

4. Patient Empowerment and Education
- Informed Decision Making:
 - Health Literacy: Providing patients with knowledge about how
various practices interact enables them to make informed
decisions about their health journeys, promoting proactive rather
than reactive care.
 - Self-care and Agency: Encouraging patients to engage in self-
monitoring practices, such as mindfulness or stress reduction
techniques, fosters empowerment and personal responsibility for
health.

5. Research and Innovation

- Development of New Therapies:
 - Clinical Studies and Trials: Conducting research to explore the
efficacy of Ayurvedic remedies alongside modern treatments can
lead to new therapeutic innovations and the validation of
traditional practices through scientific methods.
 - Expansion of Evidence Base: Systematic research can provide
the evidence needed to integrate Ayurvedic principles into
mainstream health policies and practices, influencing future
healthcare models.

6. Encouragement of Mind-Body Healing
- Addressing Comprehensive Health Needs:
  - Emphasizing Well-being: Integrative healthcare acknowledges the importance of mental and emotional health equally with physical health, promoting therapies like yoga, meditation, and counseling to treat the patient holistically.
  - Cognitive and Emotional Support: Applying Ayurvedic knowledge on subtle energies (sattva, rajas, tamas) alongside psychological theories aids in fostering mental clarity and emotional resilience.

The opportunities for integrating traditional Ayurvedic practices with modern medical diagnostics and treatments represent an exciting frontier in healthcare. This approach aligns with the growing demand for holistic, personalized, and patient-centered care, emphasizing both prevention and healing. As practitioners and researchers collaboratively explore and validate these integrated systems, they pave the way for innovative treatments and improved patient outcomes. This fusion of methodologies honors the depth of ancient traditions while embracing the precision of contemporary science, ultimately enhancing the quality of care in a diverse healthcare landscape.

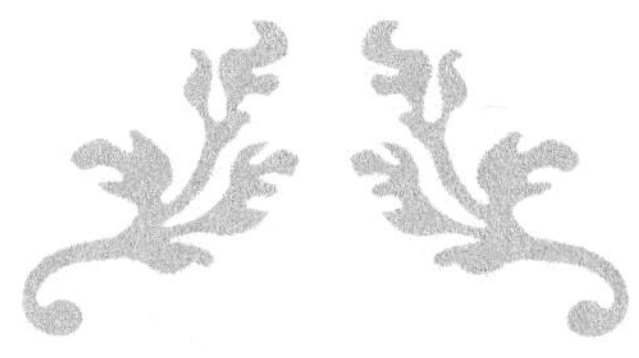

CHAPTER 8 – TRAINING AND SKILL DEVELPOMENT

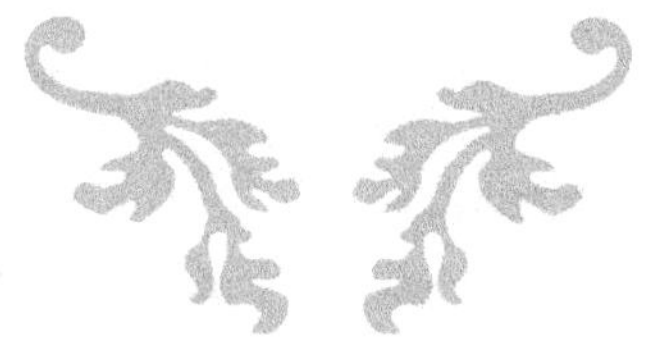

8.1 Path to Becoming a Nadi Vaidya (Pulse Expert)

Becoming a Nadi Vaidya, or a pulse expert, is a journey that requires dedication, extensive study, and practical experience. A Nadi Vaidya possesses a deep understanding of the principles of Ayurveda, particularly those related to Nadi Parikshan (pulse diagnosis), and applies this knowledge to assess and balance the doshas—Vata, Pitta, and Kapha—in patients. This path combines traditional learning with modern insights, fostering the expertise needed to excel in this specialized field.

Steps to Becoming a Nadi Vaidya

1. Foundational Education in Ayurveda
- Pursue Formal Education:
  - Enrol in a Bachelor of Ayurvedic Medicine and Surgery (BAMS) program or equivalent, depending on the country. This comprehensive education includes foundational knowledge of Ayurvedic principles, anatomy, physiology, and the identification of doshas and their functions.

- Understand Classical Texts:
  - Study key Ayurvedic texts such as the Charaka Samhita, Sushruta Samhita, and Ashtanga Hridayam. These texts offer insights into traditional diagnostic methods, including Nadi Parikshan.

2. Specialized Training in Nadi Parikshan
- Advanced Courses and Workshops:

- Enroll in specialized courses focusing on pulse diagnosis. These programs are often offered by esteemed Ayurvedic institutions or under the guidance of experienced Nadi Vaidyas and cover techniques for identifying doshic imbalances through the pulse.

- Mentorship and Apprenticeship:
  - Seek opportunities to apprentice with a seasoned Nadi Vaidya. Hands-on experience and mentorship are crucial for learning the nuances of pulse reading and developing the intuitive skills necessary for expertise.

3. Developing Practical Skills
- Extensive Practice:
  - Regularly practice pulse diagnosis on a wide range of individuals to discern subtle variations and improve diagnostic accuracy. This practice helps enhance sensitivity to different pulse qualities related to specific conditions and imbalances.

- Case Studies and Documentation:
  - Analyze and document case studies detailing pulse findings and correlating them with patient symptoms and outcomes. This practice contributes to building a personal database of experiences and enhancing diagnostic precision.

4. Integration with Modern Diagnostic Techniques
- Stay Informed on Medical Advancements:
  - Learn about modern diagnostic technologies and research that complement Nadi Parikshan. Understanding correlations between Ayurvedic diagnostics and contemporary health parameters enriches the overall diagnostic process.

- Collaborative Approach:
  - Work alongside practitioners from other disciplines, such as allopathic medicine, to integrate pulse diagnosis within a broader healthcare framework, encouraging a holistic approach to patient care.

5. Continuous Learning and Professional Development
- Attend Seminars and Conferences:
  - Engage with ongoing education by attending seminars, conferences, and symposiums related to Ayurveda and pulse diagnosis. Networking with peers and experts promotes knowledge exchange and professional growth.

- Contribute to Research:
  - Participate in or initiate research projects that explore pulse diagnosis techniques, efficacy, and integration with other diagnostic methods. Contributions to academic publications and studies help advance the field.

6. Emphasize Communication and Care
- Patient Interaction:
  - Develop strong communication skills to effectively convey diagnostic findings and treatment plans to patients. A compassionate approach is essential for fostering trust and encouraging compliance.

- Personalized Treatment Plans:
  - Utilize pulse findings to create individualized treatment plans, incorporating lifestyle modifications, dietary adjustments, and herbal therapies tailored to the specific needs of each patient.

The path to becoming a Nadi Vaidya is both challenging and rewarding, requiring a blend of traditional mastery and modern integration. By committing to lifelong learning, practical application, and patient-centered care, aspiring Nadi Vaidyas can develop the expertise needed to excel in pulse diagnosis and contribute meaningfully to the field of holistic health. This journey reflects the core principles of Ayurveda, emphasizing balance, individualized therapy, and the profound connection between practitioner and patient.

8.2 Educational Resources and Training Programs

For those aspiring to become a Nadi Vaidya, accessing the right educational resources and training programs is crucial. These programs provide the foundational and advanced knowledge necessary to master Ayurveda and Nadi Parikshan (pulse diagnosis). Here's an overview of the educational pathways and resources available for individuals interested in this specialized field.

Formal Education in Ayurveda

1. Bachelor of Ayurvedic Medicine and Surgery (BAMS):

   - Overview: This is a professional degree in Ayurveda offered by many universities and recognized Ayurvedic colleges, primarily in India and countries where Ayurveda is practiced extensively.

   - Curriculum: Includes in-depth study of Sanskrit, Ayurvedic fundamentals, anatomy, pharmacology, pathology, and diagnostic techniques, including an introduction to pulse diagnosis.

2. Postgraduate and Doctoral Programs:

- MD (Ayurveda): Postgraduate specialization programs, such as Kayachikitsa (General Medicine), often provide advanced training in diagnostic techniques, including pulse reading.

- PhD Programs: Opportunities for research-focused careers, exploring specific aspects of Ayurveda, including pulse diagnosis methodologies and their applications.

Specialized Training in Nadi Parikshan

1. Workshops and Seminars:

- These are often conducted by experienced Nadi Vaidyas, Ayurvedic practitioners, and institutes. They focus on hands-on training and cover different pulse qualities, interpretation techniques, and case studies.

2. Short Courses and Certifications:

- Offered by various Ayurvedic schools worldwide, these courses provide concentrated, in-depth training on Nadi Parikshan, suitable for practitioners who already have a foundational understanding of Ayurveda.

Renowned Institutions and Training Centres

1. Institute of Ayurveda and Integrative Medicine (I-AIM), India:

- Provides training and research opportunities related to various aspects of Ayurveda, including diagnostic practices like pulse reading.

2. The Ayurvedic Institute, USA:

- Offers comprehensive Ayurvedic training programs that include modules on traditional diagnostic methods and may cover pulse diagnosis depending on the program level.

3. Patanjali Ayurvedic College and Research Centre, India:
  - Offers BAMS and postgraduate courses with a focus on integrating traditional Ayurvedic knowledge with modern medical practices.

4. European Institute of Vedic Studies:
  - Provides online and on-site courses with workshops focused on Ayurvedic healing practices, potentially covering pulse diagnosis techniques.

Online Resources and Research Publications
1. Online Courses:
  - Platforms like Coursera, Udemy, or specific Ayurvedic schools may offer introductory courses in Ayurveda that include aspects of diagnostic techniques.

2. Research Journals and Articles:
  - Publications such as the Journal of Ayurveda and Integrative Medicine (JAIM) often publish articles related to diagnostic techniques, including pulse diagnosis, offering insights into contemporary research and developments.

3. Books and Texts:
  - Foundational Ayurvedic texts such as the Charaka Samhita and Sushruta Samhita, along with modern books on Ayurveda and pulse diagnosis, serve as valuable resources for deepening one's understanding.

Learning from Experienced Practitioners

- Mentoring and Apprenticeship:

- Shadowing experienced Nadi Vaidyas provides valuable hands-on learning opportunities beyond formal education. This apprenticeship model allows for personalized instruction and real-world experience.

- Professional Associations:
  - Joining Ayurvedic professional organizations can provide networking opportunities, access to additional training resources, and platforms for collaborative learning.

The pathway to becoming a skilled Nadi Vaidya is supported by a variety of educational resources and training programs, from formal degree courses to specialized workshops and online learning opportunities. Engaging with these resources enables aspiring practitioners to develop the expertise needed to excel in pulse diagnosis and contribute effectively to the field of holistic healthcare. By combining academic study with practical experience under expert guidance, individuals can embark on a rewarding journey of fostering health and well-being through the ancient art of Nadi Parikshan.

8.3 Ethical Considerations in Pulse Diagnosis

Pulse diagnosis, or Nadi Parikshan, is a profound and sensitive technique within Ayurveda that requires a high level of expertise, discretion, and ethical integrity. As practitioners engage in this diagnostic practice, they are entrusted with the delicate task of interpreting an individual's health through the subtle nuances of the pulse. Ethical considerations are paramount to ensuring that this practice is conducted with respect, professionalism, and patient-centered care.

Core Ethical Considerations

1. Informed Consent and Communication

- Obtaining Consent:

  - Before conducting pulse diagnosis, practitioners must obtain informed consent from the patient. This involves explaining the procedure, its purpose, and potential outcomes in a manner that the patient understands, ensuring voluntary participation.

- Transparent Communication:

  - Clear and honest communication about findings and recommendations is necessary. Practitioners should use language that is accessible and avoid technical jargon that might confuse or mislead the patient.

2. Privacy and Confidentiality

- Respecting Privacy:

  - Pulse diagnosis requires physical touch, typically involving the patient's wrist. Practitioners should ensure that the process always respects the patient's personal space and comfort levels.

- Maintaining Confidentiality:

  - All information obtained through pulse diagnosis, including health insights and personal data, must be treated as confidential. Practitioners should safeguard this information and avoid unauthorized disclosure.

3. Accuracy and Honesty in Diagnosis

- Honest Assessment:

  - Practitioners must provide truthful and accurate interpretations of pulse findings. They should avoid overstating their diagnostic capabilities or making unfounded claims about their findings.

- Acknowledging Limitations:

 - Recognize the limitations of pulse diagnosis and refrain from using it as the sole basis for diagnosing serious medical conditions. Complementary diagnostic methods should be employed when needed, and referrals to other healthcare professionals should be made as appropriate.

4. Professional Competence and Continuous Learning
- Maintaining Competence:

 - Practitioners should only perform pulse diagnosis within the limits of their training and expertise. Continuous education and training are essential to stay updated with the latest developments and to refine diagnostic skills.

- Ethical Training:

 - Training programs and institutions must instill a strong ethical foundation in practitioners, emphasizing the importance of integrity, compassion, and professionalism in pulse diagnosis.

5. Non-Discrimination and Respect for Diversity
- Cultural Sensitivity:

 - Practitioners should respect the diverse cultural, religious, and personal values of their patients. Sensitivity to cultural variations in health beliefs and practices is essential.

- Non-Discrimination:

 - All patients deserve equitable treatment regardless of their background, ethnicity, gender, or socioeconomic status. Discrimination in any form is unethical and must be actively opposed.

6. Patient Empowerment and Autonomy

- Empowering Patients:

 - Encourage patient involvement in their health journey by providing insights that empower them to make informed decisions about their care. Education on lifestyle modifications and preventive practices is a key aspect of patient empowerment.

- Respecting Autonomy:

 - Honor the patient's autonomy in making healthcare decisions. The diagnostic insights should facilitate conversations about health without imposing the practitioner's own beliefs or recommendations.

Ethical considerations are fundamental to the practice of Nadi Parikshan, guiding practitioners to engage in pulse diagnosis with integrity, respect, and professionalism. By upholding these ethical principles, practitioners not only ensure the provision of high-quality care but also foster trust and respect in the patient-practitioner relationship. This ethical framework supports Ayurveda's holistic approach, emphasizing care that is respectful, compassionate, and centered on the well-being and autonomy of each individual.

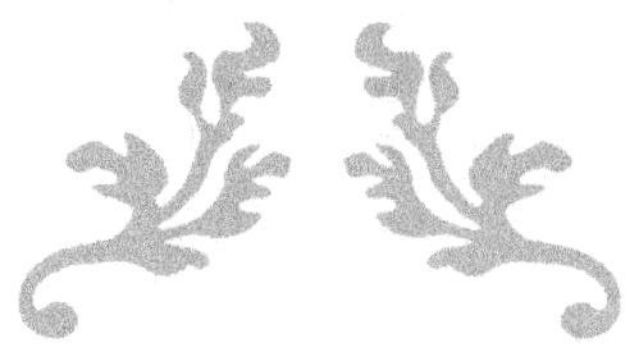

Chapter 9 – Future Directions and Research in Nadi Parikshan

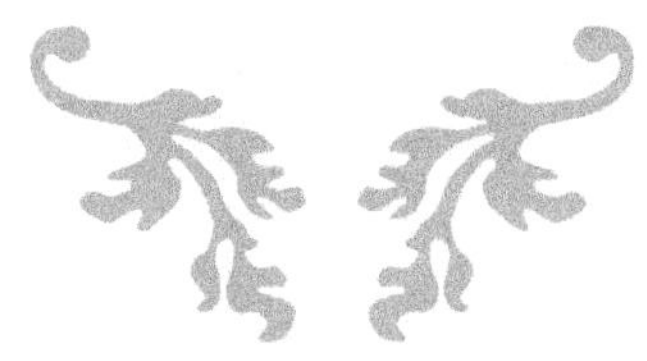

9.1 Current Research Trends in Nadi Parikshan

Nadi Parikshan, the traditional Ayurvedic practice of pulse diagnosis, is gaining attention in contemporary research as scholars and practitioners seek to validate and enhance its diagnostic potential. The integration of traditional wisdom with modern scientific methods offers valuable opportunities to deepen our understanding of Nadi Parikshan and its applications in healthcare. Here are some current research trends in this field:

1. Validation and Standardization
- Objective Measures:
  - Researchers are developing quantitative methods to objectively measure pulse characteristics that have traditionally been assessed subjectively by practitioners. This involves creating algorithms and technologies that can capture and analyze pulse waveforms, potentially reducing variability in diagnosis.

- Standardized Protocols:
  - Efforts are being made to establish standardized protocols for pulse diagnosis to ensure consistency and reliability across different practitioners and settings. Such protocols can enhance the credibility and acceptance of Nadi Parikshan in broader healthcare contexts.

2. Technological Integration
- Digital Pulse Diagnosis Tools:
  - The development of digital tools like sensors and smartphone applications aims to assist practitioners in diagnosing doshic imbalances by measuring pulse rate, rhythm, and other

parameters. These tools offer potential for increased accessibility and precision in Ayurvedic diagnostics.

- Artificial Intelligence and Machine Learning:
  - AI and machine learning technologies are being explored to analyze complex pulse data, identify patterns, and predict health outcomes. These approaches could enhance the diagnostic capabilities of Nadi Parikshan by integrating large datasets and drawing more accurate, data-driven conclusions.

3. Comparative Studies with Modern Medicine
- Correlational Studies:
  - Comparative studies are being conducted to correlate findings from Nadi Parikshan with modern diagnostic methods, such as blood tests, imaging, and cardiovascular assessments. These studies seek to reinforce the validity of traditional methods through scientific correlation with biomedical parameters.

- Integrative Health Models:
  - Research is exploring the implementation of integrative health models that combine Ayurvedic pulse diagnosis with conventional medical diagnostics. This multidisciplinary approach aims to offer more comprehensive patient assessments and improved healthcare outcomes.

4. Clinical Efficacy and Applications
- Clinical Trials and Studies:
  - Clinical trials are being undertaken to evaluate the efficacy of treatments guided by Nadi Parikshan, looking at various health conditions and patient populations. These studies aim to provide evidence for the diagnostic and therapeutic benefits of pulse assessment.

- Personalized Treatment Outcomes:
  - Research is focusing on the impact of pulse-based personalized treatment plans on patient outcomes, assessing how tailored interventions based on pulse diagnosis can influence health and healing processes.

5. Educational Research and Practitioner Training
- Training Methodologies:
  - Research into effective training methodologies for teaching Nadi Parikshan is ongoing, aiming to develop educational frameworks that enhance practitioner competence and diagnostic accuracy.

- Curriculum Development:
  - Efforts are being made to integrate modern research findings into Ayurvedic education curricula, ensuring that upcoming practitioners are equipped with both traditional knowledge and contemporary scientific insights.

6. Global Perspectives and Cross-cultural Studies
- Cross-Cultural Integration:
  - Researchers are examining the adaptation and application of Nadi Parikshan across different cultures and healthcare systems, seeking to understand its universal applicability and potential synergy with various traditional diagnostic methods.

The current research trends in Nadi Parikshan highlight a vibrant and evolving field that seeks to bridge the gap between ancient Ayurveda and modern science. By validating and refining pulse diagnosis through innovative technologies, clinical studies, and interdisciplinary approaches, researchers are working to enhance its role in contemporary healthcare. These efforts reflect a broader movement towards integrated health models that harmonize traditional wisdom with scientific advancements, aiming to deliver more holistic and effective healthcare solutions globally.

9.2 Collaborations with Scientific Communities

Collaborations between Ayurvedic practitioners and modern scientific communities are pivotal in bridging the ancient wisdom of Nadi Parikshan with contemporary medical research and practice. These collaborations aim to validate traditional practices through scientific inquiry, enhance the credibility and integration of Ayurvedic diagnostics in mainstream healthcare, and foster innovation in diagnostic techniques and treatment strategies.

Key Areas of Collaboration

1. Interdisciplinary Research Projects
- Collaborative Research Initiatives:
  - Joint research projects between Ayurvedic institutions and scientific labs allow for the exploration of pulse diagnosis using scientific methodologies. These projects often focus on the physiological correlates of pulse characteristics and their relationship with health conditions.

- Clinical Studies and Trials:
  - Collaborative clinical trials assess the efficacy of treatments guided by pulse diagnosis. By involving scientific communities,

these studies ensure rigor and validity, providing empirical evidence to support traditional diagnostic approaches.

2. Technological Development and Innovation
- Development of Diagnostic Tools:
  - Engineers and computer scientists work alongside Ayurvedic practitioners to develop and refine digital pulse diagnosis tools. These technologies aim to accurately measure and analyze pulse parameters, combining traditional insights with modern precision.

- Integration of AI and Machine Learning:
  - Collaborations focus on leveraging AI and machine learning to process large volumes of pulse data. These technologies can help identify patterns and predict health outcomes, enhancing the diagnostic potential of Nadi Parikshan.

3. Educational Partnerships
- Curriculum Development:
  - Joint efforts in developing educational curricula that incorporate both traditional Ayurvedic principles and scientific research findings help prepare practitioners who can navigate both worlds effectively.

- Training Programs and Workshops:
  - Partnerships offer training programs and workshops that focus on interdisciplinary learning, enabling practitioners from different backgrounds to gain exposure to Ayurvedic diagnostic techniques and their scientific validation.

4. Publications and Conferences

- Co-authored Publications:
  - Collaborative writing of academic papers and research articles allows for the dissemination of findings that highlight the integration of Nadi Parikshan and modern scientific methods, contributing to the body of knowledge in both fields.

- Joint Conferences and Symposiums:
  - Organizing and participating in conferences where experts from Ayurveda and scientific communities present their findings fosters dialogue, networking, and sharing of innovative ideas and best practices.

5. Global Health Initiatives
- Integrative Health Programs:
  - Partnerships in global health initiatives facilitate the inclusion of Nadi Parikshan in comprehensive healthcare models, combining traditional and modern approaches to address global health challenges.

- Cross-cultural Studies:
  - Collaborative studies that explore the application of pulse diagnosis across diverse cultural contexts help understand its universal applicability and enhance its integration into global healthcare systems.

Impact and Future Directions

Enhancing Credibility and Acceptance
- Collaborative efforts contribute significantly to increasing the credibility and acceptance of Ayurvedic practices like Nadi Parikshan in mainstream medical communities. By

demonstrating efficacy through scientific validation, these partnerships pave the way for wider acceptance and implementation of integrated healthcare approaches.

Innovative Solutions and Healthcare Integration
- The fusion of traditional knowledge with scientific advancements can lead to innovative diagnostic and therapeutic solutions, enhancing patient care. Integrated healthcare models that leverage both traditional and modern practices can offer more comprehensive and effective treatment options.

Collaborations with scientific communities represent a critical pathway for advancing the practice of Nadi Parikshan and other Ayurvedic diagnostic methods. By jointly exploring and validating traditional practices through rigorous scientific inquiry and technological innovation, these collaborations hold the promise of enriching global healthcare landscapes, ultimately fostering a more inclusive, effective, and holistic approach to health and well-being.

9.3 Innovations in Pulse Diagnosis Techniques

The field of pulse diagnosis, rooted in traditional practices like Nadi Parikshan in Ayurveda, is witnessing significant innovations driven by advancements in technology and a deeper scientific understanding. These innovations aim to enhance the accuracy, reproducibility, and accessibility of pulse diagnosis, bridging ancient wisdom with modern healthcare needs. Here are some key developments and innovations in pulse diagnosis techniques:

Technological Advancements

1. Digital Pulse Sensing and Analysis
- Wearable Devices:

 - Development of wearable tech that continuously monitors pulse characteristics, providing real-time data on heart rate, rhythm, and other vital signs. These devices use sensors such as photoplethysmography (PPG) to detect blood volume changes and offer ongoing health insights.

- Smartphone Integration:

 - Apps and smartphone attachments are being designed to allow users to perform pulse analysis independently. These technologies harness phone cameras and sensors to measure pulse waveforms, making pulse diagnosis more accessible.

2. Use of Artificial Intelligence (AI) and Machine Learning
- Pattern Recognition Algorithms:

 - AI algorithms are being designed to analyze complex pulse data, identifying patterns and deviations that may correlate with specific health conditions. These tools can enhance diagnostic precision and provide predictive analytics for health outcomes.

- Data-Driven Insights:

 - Machine learning models process large datasets to improve the interpretation of pulse characteristics, potentially leading to the development of new diagnostic markers and personalized treatment recommendations.

Enhancements in Diagnostic Techniques

1. Multi-Parameter Pulse Analysis

- Comprehensive Monitoring:

 - Modern tools analyze multiple parameters, such as pulse rate, variability, strength, and waveforms, to provide a holistic picture of cardiovascular and systemic health. This multi-faceted approach aims to mirror the holistic insights of traditional pulse diagnosis.

- Pulse Wave Velocity Measurement:

 - Innovations include non-invasive devices that measure pulse wave velocity, an indicator of arterial stiffness and cardiovascular health, offering additional insights into vascular conditions.

 2. Standardization and Calibration
- Standardized Protocols:

 - Efforts are being made to develop standardized methods for pulse measurement and interpretation, ensuring consistency and reliability across different settings and practitioners.

- Calibration Tools:

 - Calibration tools and procedures are being established to ensure that digital and AI-based pulse diagnosis devices provide accurate and reliable data.

Integration with Holistic Health Practices

1. Complementary Diagnostics:
- Interdisciplinary Approaches:

 - Integrating pulse diagnosis innovations with other diagnostic methods such as biomarker analysis, genomic data, and imaging can offer a more comprehensive understanding of health and disease.

- Cross-Disciplinary Research:
  - Collaborative research efforts are focusing on combining insights from traditional practices with modern science, leading to integrative diagnostic solutions that respect and utilize diverse medical paradigms.

2. Personalized Health Monitoring:
- Tailored Interventions:
  - Technology-backed pulse diagnosis can support personalized medicine approaches, tailoring interventions based on detailed individual health profiles and dynamic health data.

- Preventive Healthcare:
  - Continuous monitoring and early detection of anomalies allow for timely preventive measures, aligning with both traditional preventive practices and modern preventive medicine strategies.

Innovations in pulse diagnosis techniques are transforming an ancient art into a scientifically validated and technologically accessible practice. By embracing digital advancements, AI integration, and interdisciplinary research, pulse diagnosis is poised to offer enhanced diagnostic capabilities and personalized health insights. These innovations present exciting opportunities for advancing individualized care, preventive health strategies, and the broader integration of traditional wisdom with contemporary medical science, ultimately benefiting global healthcare practices.

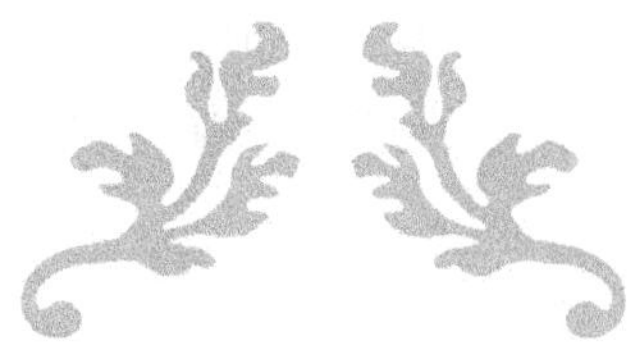

APPENDICES

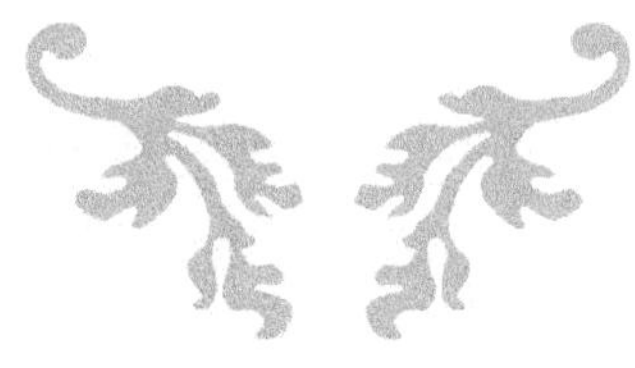

Glossary of Ayurveda Terms

A

1. **Agni**: Digestive fire responsible for digestion and metabolism.
2. **Ama**: Toxins formed due to improper digestion.
3. **Abhyanga**: Oil massage therapy to promote health and relaxation.
4. **Ahara**: Food or diet.
5. **Anuloma**: Practices or herbs that regulate proper downward movement of bodily energies.
6. **Ayurveda**: Ancient Indian science of life and holistic medicine.
7. **Ashwagandha**: A rejuvenating herb used for stress and vitality.
8. **Arishta**: Herbal fermented liquid medicine.
9. **Anjana**: Ayurvedic eye treatment using medicated eye salve.
10. **Arjuna**: A tree used for cardiac health.

B

11. **Basti**: Medicated enema, a part of Panchakarma therapy.
12. **Bala**: Strength or immunity.
13. **Bhumi**: Earth element in the Panchamahabhutas (five great elements).
14. **Bhavana**: Repeated soaking and drying of herbs to enhance potency.
15. **Brahmi**: Herb known for boosting memory and mental clarity.
16. **Bhedana**: Herbs or therapies used for expelling doshas from the body.

17. **Bhasma**: Ash of herbs or metals used in medicines.

18. **Bilva**: Bael tree, used for digestive health.

19. **Bhrajaka Pitta**: Subdosha of Pitta responsible for skin health.

20. **Bhuta Vidya**: Branch of Ayurveda dealing with psychological disorders.

C

21. **Chakra**: Energy centers in the body.

22. **Churna**: Herbal powders used in medicines.

23. **Charaka Samhita**: Ancient Ayurvedic text written by Charaka.

24. **Chikitsa**: Treatment or therapy.

25. **Chyawanprash**: Herbal formulation used as a rejuvenative tonic.

26. **Chaturbhadra**: A blend of four potent spices.

27. **Chitraka**: Herb used to kindle digestive fire.

28. **Chedana**: Therapy for expelling kapha or phlegm from the body.

29. **Chapalata**: Mental instability or restlessness.

30. **Chaturanga**: Fourfold approach to treatment: ahara, vihara, aushadha, and manasika shuddhi.

D

31. **Dosha**: Three fundamental bodily bio-energies: Vata, Pitta, Kapha.

32. **Dhaatu**: Seven tissues of the body.

33. **Dhanvantari**: Hindu deity associated with Ayurveda.

34. **Dhara**: Continuous pouring of medicated liquid on the body.

35. **Dhoopana**: Fumigation therapy for disinfection.

36. **Dhyana**: Meditation for mental and spiritual well-being.
37. **Dravya**: Substance or drug used in treatment.
38. **Draksha**: Grapes, used in Ayurveda for cooling and rejuvenation.
39. **Dashamoola**: A group of ten roots used for treating inflammation.
40. **Danti**: Plant used for purgation therapy.

E

41. **Ekadasha**: A special time for fasting and purification.
42. **Ela**: Cardamom, used for digestion and respiratory health.
43. **Eshana**: Desire or longing, important in Ayurvedic psychology.
44. **Eka-doshaja**: Disorders caused by a single dosha imbalance.
45. **Eka-mula**: Root cause of disease.

G

46. **Ghrita**: Medicated ghee used in treatments.
47. **Guggulu**: Resin used for joint health and weight management.
48. **Gandusha**: Oil pulling therapy for oral health.
49. **Guduchi**: Herb known for its immune-boosting properties.
50. **Garbhini Paricharya**: Care for pregnant women in Ayurveda.

H

51. **Hridya**: Herbs beneficial for heart health.
52. **Haritaki**: Fruit used for detoxification and rejuvenation.

53. **Hina**: Deficiency or imbalance.
54. **Hima**: Cold infusion therapy.
55. **Hridroga**: Diseases of the heart.

J

56. **Jatharagni**: Digestive fire in the stomach.
57. **Jala**: Water, one of the five elements.
58. **Jivaniya**: Herbs that provide vitality and life force.
59. **Jyotishmati**: Herb used for improving cognitive function.
60. **Jirna**: Digested or old.

K

61. **Kapha**: One of the three doshas responsible for stability and lubrication.
62. **Kshira**: Milk, often used in Ayurvedic preparations.
63. **Karma**: Actions, including therapeutic procedures.
64. **Kashaya**: Astringent taste or decoction.
65. **Karna Puranam**: Pouring medicated oil into the ears.

L

66. **Langhana**: Fasting or lightening therapy.
67. **Lepa**: Herbal paste applied to the skin.
68. **Lodhra**: Herb used for skin health and bleeding disorders.
69. **Lavanga**: Clove, used for digestion and oral health.
70. **Lekhana**: Scraping therapy to remove excess fat or toxins.

M

71. **Manas**: Mind considered integral to health.
72. **Marma**: Vital points in the body.
73. **Madhura**: Sweet taste, one of the six rasas.

74. **Mahagni**: Strong digestive fire.

75. **Mukhalepa**: Facial treatment using herbal paste.

N

76. **Nadi**: Channels or pathways for energy flow.

77. **Nasya**: Nasal administration of medicines.

78. **Nirama**: State of being free from toxins (ama).

79. **Neem**: Herb used for skin health and detoxification.

80. **Neti**: Nasal cleansing technique.

P

81. **Pitta**: Dosha responsible for digestion and metabolism.

82. **Prakriti**: Individual's constitution or body type.

83. **Panchakarma**: Five detoxification therapies.

84. **Prana**: Life force or vital energy.

85. **Pathya**: Wholesome diet and lifestyle.

R

86. **Rasa**: Taste or essence.

87. **Rakta**: Blood, one of the dhatus.

88. **Rasayana**: Rejuvenation therapy for longevity.

89. **Roga**: Disease or ailment.

90. **Raktamokshana**: Bloodletting therapy.

S

91. **Sattva**: Quality of purity and clarity of the mind.

92. **Shirodhara**: Pouring oil on the forehead for relaxation.

93. **Shilajit**: Mineral pitch used for rejuvenation.

94. **Sneha**: Oleation or use of oils.

95. **Swedana**: Fomentation or sweat-inducing therapy.

96. **Tridosha**: The three doshas: Vata, Pitta, Kapha.
97. **Taila**: Oil used in treatments.
98. **Tikta**: Bitter taste, one of the six rasas.
99. **Triphala**: Herbal combination of three fruits for detoxification.
100. **Twak**: Skin, a vital organ in Ayurveda.

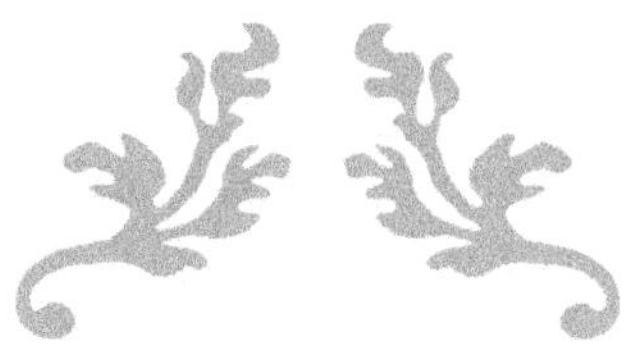

REFERENCES

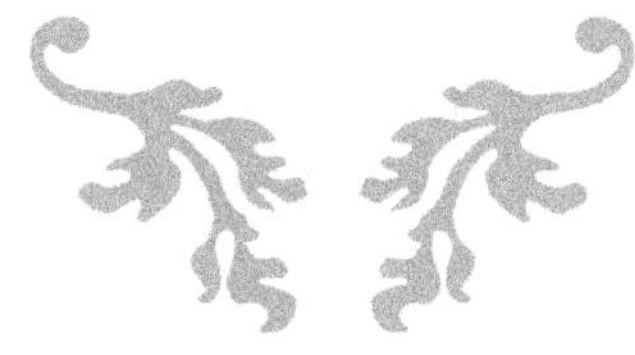

References of the Nadi Parikshana in ancient Indian Text

Nadi Parikshana (pulse diagnosis) is an integral part of Ayurvedic diagnostics. While the classical Ayurvedic texts do not have a dedicated or exclusive treatise solely focused on Nadi Parikshana, references to pulse examination and related principles are scattered across several classical Ayurvedic works. Here are the key texts and their references:

1. Charaka Samhita

- **Author**: Acharya Charaka
- **Relevance**: While Charaka does not explicitly discuss Nadi Parikshana as a primary diagnostic tool, he emphasizes the importance of examining the doshas, dhatus, and malas to understand the prakriti and vikriti (nature and imbalance) of the patient.
- **References**:
    - Chapter: **Vimana Sthana** (Examination methods)
    - Key Concept: Clinical examination of disease through observation, palpation, and questioning.

2. Sushruta Samhita

- **Author**: Acharya Sushruta
- **Relevance**: Focuses on examination techniques, especially touch and palpation, which are foundational to Nadi Parikshana.
- **References**:
    - Chapter: **Sharira Sthana** (Study of the body)

- o Key Concept: Descriptions of pulse in the context of blood circulation and vitiated doshas.

3. Ashtanga Hridaya

- **Author**: Vagbhata
- **Relevance**: Provides comprehensive guidelines for diagnostic approaches, including tactile methods that relate to pulse diagnosis.
- **References**:
  - o Chapter: **Sutra Sthana** (Basic Principles)
  - o Key Concept: Examination of the body and doshas through sensory modalities, including touch.

4. Bhavaprakasha

- **Author**: Bhavamishra
- **Relevance**: Contains detailed diagnostic insights, including indirect mentions of pulse characteristics.
- **References**:
  - o Focus on recognizing dosha imbalances through physical signs, indirectly pointing to pulse examination.

5. Sharangadhara Samhita

- **Author**: Sharangadhara
- **Relevance**: One of the most significant texts explicitly mentioning and elaborating on Nadi Parikshana.
- **References**:
  - o Chapter: **Purva Khanda (First Section)**

o   Key Concept: Detailed descriptions of pulse characteristics corresponding to the tridoshas (Vata, Pitta, Kapha) and their combinations.

o   Considered the foundational text for later advancements in Nadi Parikshana.

6. Yoga Ratnakara

- **Author**: Unknown (Composed by later Ayurvedic scholars)
- **Relevance**: A comprehensive work with elaborate descriptions of pulse examination and its correlation with doshas and diseases.
- **References**:
    - o   Chapter: **Nadi Vigyana**
    - o   Key Concept: Detailed insights into interpreting pulse in various health conditions.

7. Basavarajeeyam

- **Author**: Basavaraj
- **Relevance**: A lesser-known but significant work focusing on Nadi Parikshana.
- **References**:
    - o   Chapter: **Nadi Lakshana**
    - o   Key Concept: Analysis of the qualities of pulse and their diagnostic implications.

8. Hatha Yoga Pradipika

- **Author**: Swatmarama
- **Relevance**: Though primarily a yogic text, it contains references to pranic flows, which are foundational for understanding pulse rhythms in Ayurveda.

10. Kashyapa Samhita

- **Author**: Acharya Kashyapa
- **Relevance**: Primarily a pediatric (Kaumarbhritya) text, but it briefly mentions physical and tactile examination methods relevant to pulse examination in identifying disorders in children and their dosha imbalances.

11. Bhela Samhita

- **Author**: Acharya Bhela (Disciple of Punarvasu Atreya)
- **Relevance**: An ancient Ayurvedic text parallel to Charaka Samhita, providing insights into the observation of bodily functions. While the text does not directly elaborate on pulse diagnosis, it focuses on the detailed examination of prakriti (constitution) and dosha interactions, foundational to understanding pulse.

12. Madhava Nidana

- **Author**: Madhavakara
- **Relevance**: Primarily a text on pathology (Nidana), Madhava Nidana emphasizes diagnostic techniques to identify the root cause of diseases, including indirect allusions to pulse examination in relation to doshas and systemic conditions.
- **Key Sections**:
  - **Nidana Sthana**: Diagnosis of systemic disorders.

13. Bhavaprakasha Nighantu (Materia Medica)

- **Author**: Bhavamishra
- **Relevance**: Contains references to herbs and formulations that affect doshas, indirectly influencing

pulse diagnosis by aligning specific herbs with observed dosha states.

---

14. Harita Samhita

- **Author**: Sage Harita
- **Relevance**: Contains descriptions of diagnostic methods, including the indirect mention of tactile assessment and energy flow analysis, which relate to Nadi Parikshana.

---

15. Rasa Ratna Samuchchaya

- **Author**: Unknown
- **Relevance**: This text focuses on Rasashastra (alchemy and herbo-mineral preparations) but also includes references to clinical examination techniques, including Nadi Pariksha, as part of understanding dosha states before administering rasayana therapies.

---

16. Nadi Vijnanam (A Later Text)

- **Relevance**: A specialized text focusing entirely on Nadi Pariksha.
- **Highlights**:
  - Interpretation of doshic imbalances through pulse.
  - Detailed descriptions of Vata, Pitta, Kapha rhythms and their combinations.
  - Practical methods for identifying diseases based on pulse variations.

---

17. Nadi Darpanam

- **Author**: Mahadeva

- **Relevance**: A dedicated work on pulse diagnosis.
- **Key Insights**:
  - Describes how to evaluate the strength, rhythm, and quality of the pulse.
  - Links between pulse changes and specific diseases.

18. Hatha Ratnavali

- **Author**: Srinivasabhatta Mahayogindra
- **Relevance**: Though primarily a yogic text, it highlights prana (life force) and energy channels, foundational to understanding pulse diagnosis in a yogic and Ayurvedic framework.

19. Ananda Kanda

- **Author**: Unknown (Later compilation)
- **Relevance**: An extensive text on alchemy, with sections on body diagnostics, including Nadi Pariksha as a vital tool for identifying energy imbalances.

20. Siddha Medicine Contributions

- While not strictly Ayurveda, the Siddha tradition, closely related to Ayurveda, contains specialized texts on pulse diagnosis, including works like:
  - **Siddha Maruthuvam**: Discusses the integration of pulse analysis with tridosha and Sapta Dhatu (seven body tissues).

Additional Manuscripts and Commentaries on Nadi Pariksha

1. **Nadi Chintamani**: A later work focusing on advanced pulse diagnosis.

2. **Nadi Kaumudi**: Elaborates on subtle variations in the pulse to diagnose chronic conditions.
3. **Vasishtha Nadi Shastra**: A detailed commentary on pulse rhythms based on ancient yogic and Ayurvedic traditions.

Applications Across Ayurveda and Yoga Texts

- Many texts refer indirectly to **pranic flow** (Prana Vata), the movement of **ojas**, and the impact of these on bodily rhythms, which is core to pulse analysis.
- Commentators like **Dalhana** and **Chakrapani Datta** (on Sushruta and Charaka) expand on the importance of tactile examination in clinical diagnosis, which includes pulse examination.

Cross-Cultural and Ayurvedic-Siddha Overlaps

Many Indian medical systems, including Siddha, TCM (Traditional Chinese Medicine), and Tibetan Medicine, share roots in energy channel and pulse examination techniques. Some Ayurvedic texts like **Sharangadhara Samhita** and **Yoga Ratnakara** have influenced and been influenced by these overlapping traditions.

Recent scholarly publications have delved into **Nadi Pariksha** (pulse diagnosis), exploring its traditional methodologies and integrating modern scientific approaches. Notable works include:

1. **"Pulse (Nadi) Analysis for Disease Diagnosis: A Detailed Review"** (2022)
   This review examines the role of Nadi Pariksha in assessing diseases and psychological conditions, comparing it with

pulse analysis techniques in Traditional Chinese Medicine and Traditional Korean Medicine. It discusses the significance of the three doshas—Vata, Pitta, and Kapha—and their imbalances as indicators of disease. Springer Link

2. **"Traditional Practices and Recent Advances in Nadi Pariksha: A Comprehensive Review"** (2018)
    This comprehensive review highlights the traditional significance of Nadi Pariksha in assessing Tridoshas and various physiological and psychological states. It also discusses recent technological advancements that aim to standardize and quantify pulse diagnosis, bridging traditional practices with modern scientific methods. Unbound Medicine

3. **"Nadi Pariksha: Wrist Pulse Analysis with Traditional and Modern Techniques"** (2016)
    This article addresses the challenges of subjectivity in traditional pulse analysis and explores modern techniques and instruments developed to standardize and quantify Nadi Pariksha, enhancing its reliability in both clinical and research settings. ijapr

4. **"Review on Modern and Ayurvedic Aspects of Nadi Pariksha"** (2023)
    This review focuses on the pulse measurement sites used in Tridosha analysis, comparing traditional Nadi properties with modern pulse parameters such as pulse wave velocity and arterial stiffness. It highlights recent advances in pulse wave analysis and their relevance to Nadi Pariksha. Sanjeevani Darshan

5. **"Nadi Pariksha: An Ancient Ayurvedic Method of Diagnosis"** (2017)
    This publication delves into the historical context and methodologies of Nadi Pariksha as detailed in classical Ayurvedic texts, emphasizing its importance as a diagnostic tool in traditional medicine.